Let the Whole
Thundering World
Come Home

Also by Natalie Goldberg

Let the Whole Thundering World Come Home

A Memoir

NATALIE GOLDBERG

SHAMBHALA
Boulder · 2018

Shambhala Publications, Inc.
4720 Walnut Street
Boulder, Colorado 80301
www.shambhala.com

9 8 7 6 5 4 3 2 1

FIRST EDITION
Printed in the United States of America

⊗ This edition is printed on acid-free paper that meets the
American National Standards Institute z39.48 Standard.
♻ This book is printed on 30% postconsumer recycled paper.
For more information please visit www.shambhala.com.

Distributed in the United States by Penguin Random House LLC
and in Canada by Random House of Canada Ltd

Designed by Steve Dyer

LIBRARY OF CONGRESS CATALOGING-IN-PUBLICATION DATA
Names: Goldberg, Natalie, author.
Title: Let the whole thundering world come home: a memoir /
Natalie Goldberg.
Description: First edition. | Boulder: Shambhala, 2018.
Identifiers: LCCN 2017039916 | ISBN 9781611805673 (paperback: alk. paper)
Subjects: LCSH: Goldberg, Natalie—Health. | Cancer—Patients—Biography. |
Authors—United States—Biography. | Painters—United States—Biography.
Classification: LCC RC265.6.G65 A3 2018 |DDC 362.19699/4—dc23
LC record available at https://lccn.loc.gov/2017039916

FOR BAKSIM

With love and appreciation

Repeat

Tell me something beautiful

How sound repeats itself
The rooftops look backward
as the notes make a chorus
of voices

This fantasy number sixty-seven
How long can it go on?
How many more days can we live
in this beautiful thing?

Someday the real and unreal
will collide
The shell fall apart

There is so little time
Only poems will last
and the mountain ranges of Beethoven

So tell me something good
before it's too late

CONTENTS

PREFACE

During what I have come to call the Infusion Months of Summer—during the series of chemo infusions I had to battle the cancer raging inside me—and between the long visits to the Christus St. Vincent Regional Cancer Center, constant visits from friends, exhaustion, fever, sadness, sparks of extreme emotions, I wrote a book. Not this book but *The Great Spring*. A book that could be considered the afterword to this book.

Before I started the infusions, in the spring months when I was avoiding my cancer diagnosis, I didn't pick up a pen. I had no language for what I was going through. In March and April, I painted abstracts. In the silence of paint, color, form, I attempted to express what I didn't understand, what was way below the level of my conscious mind. When I gave in to the infusions, I began writing again.

For years I had aimed to create a particular collection of essays. Sitting on the couch in the lovely prison of my living room—when I had no energy to run around—and during long quiet afternoons when no one was there, I entered a secret island of peace. I left cancer behind and wrote about tennis and my father playing ball with me in the backyard. I collected past published essays and found new essays in my notebooks—surprising ones about being in Iowa during the 2008 presidential campaign and getting lost searching for the stone lions in the Bandelier back country. Essays that talked about how I lived my life, backed by Zen and writing; about going to Japan, France, and Archer City, Texas. That book claimed and asserted little-known parts of me. In case I died—I had no idea what the outcome of these treatments would be—at least I would have recorded times when I was alive. Maybe I wasn't always paying attention, but life—poignant corners of it—came back to me.

As I wrote, years of practice kicked in, not with my usual determination and drive, but with something more serene. In the afternoons, while healthy people were grocery shopping, running up mountains, picking up children at school, waiting for the red light to turn green, I was able to find a small victory in the center of cancer—to forget it, leave it, and do what I love. Having cancer wasn't everything, even right in the middle of having cancer. I thought of Lucian Freud, the premier British portrait painter, who died a few years ago at ninety-three, painting until the last. Death for him was like an afterthought.

• • •

The writing of this book came after cancer.

I never planned to write a book about cancer. I was on the other side and still alive, with my own aim: to wake up America through writing. And yet . . .

A saying exists: a writer gets to live twice. First we live, and then we write about what we have lived. Like a cow that brings up its feed and chews it again, a writer has a second chance to digest experience. The second time is in the notebook or in front of a computer screen. Often the second time is the real life for a writer. It is then we get to claim our existence.

At lunch a friend told me that writing about my illness was a bit crazy. "Cut your losses and go on. You're restimulating yourself."

I sat up straight in my seat, "I'm a writer. This is what writers do."

I wanted to grab a hunk of living again and hold on tight. But it wouldn't have been genuine if I skipped over what was raw, dark, and painful. Another adage a writer needs to know: the things we avoid have energy. If I ignored suffering, the life of my writing would die. You can't hold back, hide, disclaim. You have to bare your teeth and go back into the seething heat. If I didn't write this book, no other book would possibly ever come.

Besides, I wanted to know what happened to me. When I was inside the world of cancer, I was just trying to survive. Slam bam—hit by diagnoses, one after the other, that shattered any composure I ever thought I had—hospital rooms, procedures, institutions, fast decisions, medicines I never heard of before. I wanted to record this also for the reader: when you go through extreme sickness, when everything you know and lived is tossed out the window and glass shatters—I want to say *we are not crazy.* This too is part of life. Don't give up. Pay attention. We have to make ourselves larger to include the inconceivable. So many of us imagine—certainly I did—lying peacefully in our own bed during our last days, serenely bidding good-bye to relatives and friends. Good luck. It's rare.

I felt so out there alone on a ledge. I looked for and needed to hear or read what other people went through, but I could find little about the nitty-gritty experience. I wanted to record my experience as a marker for others, even though everyone's circumstances will be different.

For me this wasn't war, something to fight. Disease was another aspect of human life. Could I be in the middle of it, not so much be victorious but actually flower, become more tender, more inside human understanding? Could it open love? And reflection? Could I stand inside the storm, be drenched and endure, whether into life or into death?

In the *Book of Serenity*, an ancient Zen text from China, is case 36, "Master Ma Is Unwell." Given to us to ponder, not only with logic, but with the whole of our being.

Master Ma is sick in bed.

The monastery superintendent stops in and asks, "Master, how is your venerable state these days?"

The Great Teacher looks up and replies, "Sun face buddha, moon face buddha."

We can be awake on both sides of the coin, in sickness and in health, in light and in the dark. In both states we can glow.

Can we do this?

I called on painting, writing, and Zen to help me on my way—those three practices I used throughout my life. Would they hold me now in good stead?

At the same time that eternity swung open in front of my shocked face, my partner of five years confronted her own deep challenge. Beside me, yet separate and apart, Yu-kwan peered over the edge into the vast dark, stumbled, and was caught by another cancer, in a different part of her body. It arrived unbidden and relentless. Her cells went out of whack and grew malignant. This book is also about how we continued together and alone.

None of us gets away from carrying the genes of sickness, old age, and death. May this book help build our capacity to relate to illness and to face whatever reality we encounter.

WE WON'T LAST FOREVER

I travel all the way to Kitada, Japan, to Taizoin Temple, near the Sea of Japan, to find the ashes of my Zen teacher, Katagiri Roshi. I discover his tombstone in a row of rounded-top markers signifying his teaching lineage.

It is raining hard. I push off my hood, throw off my slicker, and prostrate myself three times on the wet earth, then kneel in front of his stone. Pushing the dripping hair from my forehead, rain running down my cheeks, I speak to my old teacher: "Took me a while, but I made it." It's been eight years since he died, and I cannot say how good I feel being near his ashes. Two rhododendron, a camellia bush, then rice paddies in the distance.

I'd heard about this place through Katagiri. For years it was only his teacher and young Katagiri, alone in the temple practicing. When Katagiri told his teacher he was going to America, the teacher said nothing, but from his teacher's back, walking behind him, young Katagiri could tell he was lonely.

In the twelve years I studied with him, for six of them I lived in a two-story duplex on Emerson Avenue six blocks from the Minnesota Zen Center and walked the back alleys at 4:45 a.m. to sit an hour each early morning in the zendo with him erect in front of the altar. I was irregular for the first years, but he was there morning after morning. "Sitting," he said, "for all sentient beings every moment forever." His dedication eventually penetrated my skin and bones. He became my great writing teacher, inspiring me to continue under all circumstances. I learned not to be tossed away by resistance, inertia, boredom, the vagaries of the human mind. In that simple building, across from Lake Calhoun in the middle of Minneapolis in the heart of the country, I touched the ground of being.

It's now been twenty-eight years since he died. Three or four times a year, I dream he has returned from the dead and is teaching again. I am always nervous and at first don't go to see him. Then I sign up for a retreat, accidentally sleep through the morning service, then grab a pink cushion and settle in.

We never actually meet again face-to-face in the dreams, but I imagine his skin—dried and darkened, pulled hard across his cheeks, the way he looked in the coffin before cremation. I wake.

What can the dead teach the living?

I'm still alive, still on the other side. His death taught me that he and I are one.

1.

I ARRIVED EARLY to a signing for my new novel. It was 1995 and I was sitting in the Taos Book Shop and chatting with Barbara Zaring, who had painted the cover to my book. Two young women poured through the door. They had just attended a palm-reading workshop and were full of exuberant knowledge. One took my friend's bony hand. "You have a happy marriage."

My friend bobbed her head up and down.

"And creative work." Then they enumerated more details I knew to be true. I was impressed.

My turn. The one with long red hair glanced down at my knuckles and tapered, small fingers. "You are very sick."

The other woman confirmed it. They didn't even turn my hand over to see my palm.

I pulled away and tucked my hands under the table.

The shadow of that long-ago dark omen was now stepping forward.

• • •

"Your doctor called and left a message," Yu-kwan sat across from me. I had just finished teaching a writing retreat in Rhinebeck, New York, where I luxuriated in afternoons telling stories to my friend Wendy on the white porch of our bunk-like rooms. Yu-kwan, my new girlfriend, lived in New York City and came up to meet me before heading to a friend's house for the weekend. While she stayed in Rhinebeck, I planned to go to her city apartment. We had just sat down at an outdoor café.

"My doctor? Why would she call?"

"She said to call her back." She handed me her phone.

I dialed. I waited for the doctor to get on the line. My lunch arrived—pizza with figs and mozzarella—and I began eating.

Eventually the doctor picked up her call, and with no pleasantries said, "There are indications you have chronic lymphocytic leukemia."

Leukemia? I managed to hear that word. I also heard the word *death*.

"They are doing further tests to verify it," she explained.

I wanted to finish the pizza and enjoy the short time I had with Yu-kwan before I dropped her off. But my tongue kept running over my doctor's words as if they were a sore tooth. *I cannot have leukemia—I don't even know for sure what it is.*

I drove that night down the Saw Mill River Parkway to Henry Hudson Parkway, made some wrong turns, and found myself in the middle of a tough area of the Bronx, almost out of gas. I had to exit. An Esso station—lively on a Friday night—was on the corner. All the gas pumps were being used; cars waited for cars to pull out; two men exited the station, each with a carton of cigarettes; a woman stood on the curb sucking a long inhale, curling her toes in a slip of sandal. The air was vibrating. I sidled slowly up to a pump behind a low car with its radio screeching hip-hop. Hip-hop doesn't screech; it bops and bobs fast. But I was screeching inside. *I might have leukemia.* I was lost and my tank was empty.

The man on the other side of the gas pump had a goatee and a blue cap on his head. I asked him, "How do I get to the Upper West Side—Manhattan?"

His face showed delight. He knew the way and could help. "Go to the second light. Make a left. Then a right at the next light. You'll see an entrance sign. . . ."

I repeated every turn once and then again.

He nodded and gave me a thumbs-up. Many times over the last years I've thought of him. To know directions is a good thing.

Almost midnight, the lights unfurling; my little rental zipped into the right lane of the curving route into the Big Apple.

I left my suitcase untouched on the dining room floor of Yu-kwan's apartment. I couldn't sleep that night. I moved from chair to chair in my rumpled clothes, never switching on a light, looking out the windows at the jazzed neon and yellow cabs, finally stripping down naked and lying on top of the sheets, staring at the ceiling, listening to the forever hum of traffic.

As a tinge of light touched the dark sky, I prayed with the slightest twist of hope that the final results would be negative.

• • •

In 1990 my Zen teacher died of lymphoma after a year in and out of hospitals and several rounds of chemo. The last weeks he lay in bed, hardly stirring. A Zen student sat with him through each night as slowly, the irreversible cold crawled through his body.

I flew into Minneapolis in late afternoon a few hours after his death. March first. The gray, brooding lake was across the street from the white, three-story Zen center. The branches of trees would be bare at least another six weeks.

He was already laid out in the *zendo*. The first dead body I'd ever seen. For three days we sat with him, until he was cremated.

I studied Zen Buddhism, but the old family religion never left me. In Judaism you bury the body within twenty-four hours. I was pushing against the mandates of my birth by sitting with a dead body for so long. I felt shattered and lost without him. We had gone deep together in the last twelve years. How do you resolve the death of someone so important to you? You don't.

Two months after Roshi died, I entered an explosive, wildly sexual love affair that continued for ten months. When we argued, I bent over and sobbed as if the earth had split open. I knew it wasn't about the relationship. Grief—long, deep, old, past this lifetime—erupted. I'd lost something huge. I was pulled in two directions—this manic ecstatic sexual scrambling versus that violent pull inside toward destruction, the end of everything.

Two months into this new relationship, I noticed three long marks behind my left ear—spider bites?—and a general weakening. I went to a doctor.

"Shingles," he pronounced.

"What's that?"

He explained it was a nerve infection that came from stress. Nothing to be done. It would go away on its own.

Something else was laying the groundwork for my sick state: the stress I carried for years from my divorce. In my early thirties, feeling invincible in my sorrow, I ate for two years—mostly chocolate croissants and chocolate chip cookies. They were baked in glorious abundance at the corner café. The odor filtered like a siren song through the room of customers hunched over newspapers and notebooks where I wrote my sorrows daily. Like my Zen teacher, the place is long defunct.

I was now, at sixty-three years old, finding out I had cancer. From the age of forty-two I had understood something was wrong with me. But no one in twenty-five years could find anything. *Maybe chronic fatigue? Maybe Epstein-Barr?* Any good doctor I'd hear about, I'd make an appointment with. "Your blood work is fine— only your white cells are a bit elevated. A recent cold or flu, probably." I'd nod, fold up my half-hopes of some ghostly cure, and leave.

Why did I think I was sick? I wrote books, hiked, taught all over the country. I was not a hypochondriac. But when I'd get the flu, as I did each winter, shot or no shot, I'd drag out of bed after five weeks, while my friends recovered in two. If something was in the air, I'd catch it. I felt at some edge, as though my immune system were so thin it was transparent.

Eventually I learned that the double stress of divorce and death made me ready for the slam punch of that disease groping its blind path into my blood and coasting through my veins for twenty-five years. It found a gaping hole in my immune system, crawled inside, and settled, inactive but patient, waiting through my forties and fifties and early sixties.

2.

ON A WEDNESDAY morning, sitting in my old blue Volvo in a parking lot after just getting a facial—my cheeks redolent with cream, all pores clean—I called the Cancer Center in Santa Fe, persuaded an oncologist to look up my chart. The oncologist I was assigned to was on vacation, and no one else was willing to give me the results of my blood tests. "Sure, I can do that," he said. He came back on the line. "It's positive for CLL."

"What?"

"Really, it's nothing. It's at zero level. It's nothing to worry about. It's no problem. Just make an appointment next week, when your doctor is back in the office."

I hung up and sat in the barren lot staring out at a brown hump of pale dirt. A white Acura pulled up next to me. I put the key in the ignition, moved into reverse, and slipped out of my spot.

What did I do the rest of the day? I don't remember. The information, like a wild animal, followed me one hundred paces behind. I tried to ignore it, numb with refusal. *This cannot be. This is not the way the world is.*

And what way, exactly, is the world? The way I wanted it to be. Death a long-distance call. I wanted to deal with death at the proper time—in my eighties or nineties.

That night I called friends while I sat in my living room in my summer cotton pajamas. I told them of my diagnosis. As soon as we hung up, many ran immediately to Google to do research.

Eddie and Mary were different. They called from a restaurant where we often ate together. "We thought we'd bring over a chocolate pot."

"No, I don't want it, but come over."

Mary repeated the offer. I normally loved that pudding.

"No, I'm really not interested."

When they came over, the late August sun was slanting on the back porch. They sat on the couch, and I sat on a chair opposite. What was there to say? Mary, who is a nurse, reminded me that the cancer was at level zero.

"Yeah, but it won't stay that way."

• • •

In 1979 a fellow Zen student was killed in the streets of San Francisco at the age of twenty-two. Katagiri Roshi's admonition: "Human beings have an idea they are fond of—that we die in old age. That's just an idea. We don't know when our death will come. Chris's death has come now."

Chris was Chris Pirsig, the son of Robert Pirsig, who wrote the well-loved *Zen and the Art of Motorcycle Maintenance*. The book was based on a trip from Minneapolis to San Francisco the author took with his young son Chris on a motorcycle. It was the middle of November when Chris was stabbed in that fatal mugging. I stood out back of the zendo during a break in the retreat after Katagiri had made his announcement. I'd never before heard a pronouncement like Roshi's—of course it was true. People died at all ages. I never forgot it until death came close to me.

Katagiri himself died young, at the age of sixty-two, one year younger than I was now.

• • •

Zen training harped on death. *We won't last forever. Wake up. Don't waste your life*. But Zen's urging seemed artistic, remote.

I was deeply aware that human beings were dying in Vietnam, then in Iraq, all over the world. One person's death was my death. I could meditate and feel the poignant, exquisite melting of boundaries, the compassion for all beings, the deathless place of interconnectedness. That was all fine. Then cancer—a nugget of death—entered my individual body. I was suddenly not connected to anything, about to disappear—forever unknown, disregarded, lost in eternity.

All I heard from people who had survived cancer was how they were victorious. I know they meant to encourage me, but it left me lonelier. I needed to hear about being in the deep pool of fear before you swim out.

The first help I received was from a woman named Sue from Boston. In the fall I went on a three-day solo retreat at a just-finished set of cabins in La Madera, north of Santa Fe. She was there because she'd helped build them. She'd been a business executive on the East Coast and fifteen years earlier had been diagnosed with breast cancer, both breasts. It turned her life upside down. She left her job and eventually joined with an old friend from Antioch College to create these glorious cabins. Her husband and kids still lived in Boston, and she commuted back and forth.

As she helped me with my luggage, I told her how scared I was. Though her cancer had been many years ago, her old fear was accessible to her. She put down the box she was carrying and trembled, telling me about her first six months of dealing with it. "Every possible test came out positive."

Her sharing helped. I didn't feel so crazy that I was so shattered.

Twice a day I recited a loving-kindness chant and meditated on the pier she had built, jutting out into a pond full of ducks. The weather was sweater warm, the light low and still full. *May I be attentive and gentle toward my own discomfort and suffering. . . . May I receive others with sympathy and understanding. . . .*

When I left, I gave Sue a copy of the chant.

I tried to find the words to describe my emotions to two or three friends. Unless I talked, no one would have any idea what I was going through. The hard part was trusting that someone would understand, when *I* didn't understand.

• • •

Sean called from Taos. "I think I know what you feel. Remember ten years ago, when I had a thyroid imbalance? The doctor came at me with a needle right at my throat. It's such a vulnerable place. I was brave, squeezing Tania's hand, but the minute he went out of the room, I began sobbing like a five-year-old. I fell apart." A pause. "Then the doctor came back. 'We have to do it again. We didn't get enough fluid.'"

I could feel Sean's shoulders shake, even on the phone. I said, "I always wondered why what happened seemed like such a big deal for you. All I knew was you had to take a pill."

3.

WE MET WITH the oncologist—me, my longtime friend Annie Lewis, and Yu-kwan, who was visiting from Manhattan. Yu-kwan wanted me to come to New York, where, she insisted, they had the best doctors and medical care. It was inconceivable for her that good doctors could be out in the boondocks of New Mexico. I told her no, I wanted someone near my home—and that New Mexico had plenty of good doctors.

"How did I get it?" I asked the oncologist.

"We don't know. Have you lived near fields that were sprayed with pesticides?"

"I don't know."

"They are doing studies along the Platte River in Nebraska. All rainwater in the area eventually runs into that river. The insecticides, the fertilizers, are carried and dumped there. It's a cancer corridor. High proportions of people living along the Platte have cancer like yours."

"I love Nebraska," I said, more interested in place than science.

She'd done further tests on my blood and determined that I also had a genetic marker, whatever that meant.

Eventually she said, "There's nothing to do at this point. Come twice a year for a checkup and blood tests."

I never went back. *Why should I?* I thought. *I'm at zero.*

• • •

For the first years of my zero-level CLL I told only a few people. Partly I just wanted the cancer to go away. Partly I was focused on a mission to spread writing practice, to show people they can trust and have a relationship with their own mind, a confidence in their own experience. It was a human right to write, to accept how we see, think, and feel.

I wanted everyone to come alive in this one great life. In my zeal, I ignored the truth of my own mortality. I couldn't face my own sickness and death, and as a result I became scratchier, tighter, more agitated in some cellular, unconscious way. And also more vulnerable—raw, right at the edge of truth.

In 2011 I was leading a writing intensive with thirty students. We met once a season for a year. Between meetings the students worked on their own. We had become close in the practice time together. We sat in meditation, did slow walking practice with mindful steps, wrote, ate in silence with each other. Below the level of social detail and constant talk, we dropped to an unspoken awareness and intimacy.

Soon after I had knowledge of my secret leukemia, the autumn gathering convened. By the middle of that week we were very much in tune. When we were practicing mindful walking in the zendo during the last two days, each time I passed Dorotea, she whispered under her breath: *Don't die, don't die.* A shiver ran the length of my spine.

Dorotea knew nothing about my medical condition, but in the extensive hours of practice, boundaries melted. We were attuned to each other's twisted agony and greatness on an unconscious level.

Each time she whispered that phrase in my presence, a long lineage of teachers vibrated through me. I did not want her—or any of my students—to suffer the way I did when Katagiri Roshi died. And I would surely go, no doubt about it, sometime, no matter what form of denial I played.

While I mostly ignored my diagnosis, not wanting to take a backward step into this new, larger truth, it showed me just how much I was in love with all of my life. I even loved the 5:00 a.m. straight-shot, hour-long drive to the Albuquerque airport through the open dry mesas; the security lines, bending down to untie shoelaces, jacket off, all back on at the other end. I loved the teaching, the students—even the difficult ones—the pen on paper. My enthusiasm often turned to sleepless nights, but still I loved the walking through exhaustion, the small bags of plane peanuts found in my purse, the tedious flights, my complaints and grievances that American students didn't read closely or care about literature. Illness or no illness, I had the energy to want more for them. Where did it come from?

I had been trained well under the guidance of Katagiri Roshi. *Jump in, no excuses. Exert the force of your life. Persevere under all circumstances.* Zen gave me the tools; the practice lit me into bright action for all sentient beings. True, we also sat stone still for many, many hours, but that stillness ignited my life force. I'd been brought up in a sleepy, conventional suburban town. The fire of practice burned up the confining cloak on my back. Zen tells us that we are already free, that we should simply become who we are, but how to do this? In that cold zendo in Minnesota I was taught how; I was given the means for action.

But still I did not yet know how to turn 180 degrees and face the unknown, the void. Cancer demanded that I let the whole thundering world come home, that I accept the horror and unknown of human life—and death. Zen taught that, too, but I was not ready to receive it.

THIS WAS MY LIFE

Carson McCullers was raised in Columbus, Georgia. I visit her home, finally made into a museum by Columbus State University. I go downtown and ask a young clerk in a pharmacy, then a saleswoman in a dress shop, if they ever read her, and they shake their heads no.

"Did you go to the local Columbus high school?"

"Yes. Never heard of her."

In Europe she is recognized along with Hemingway and Fitzgerald. Of all writers, she is most important to me. We read *The Ballad of the Sad Café* in ninth grade on Long Island in Mr. Cate's English class, and I never got over it. But she left her hometown—and a small town marks you, never forgives you for leaving, no matter how successful you become.

Also, late in her life, around the early sixties, she offered all of her papers and manuscripts to the Columbus Public Library with one stipulation: they allow negroes to use the facility. This, too, was unacceptable.

I also visit her grave in Nyack, New York, another small town, this time along the Hudson, north of the Big Apple. I often visit the graves of writers and painters I admire, to pay homage, to acknowledge where we all end, and also in case there might be a trace of them still around. I want them to know, in this tough world, that what they did mattered. It's a practice of heart, of gratitude.

Carson lived in Nyack for the last twenty years of her life, mostly sick but still writing, her work haunted by the Deep South, her mother living with her. I only find out much later—fifty years after her death—that the references to Dr. Mary Mercer, always accompanying anything I read about Carson in Nyack, were not about her being Carson's doctor but were because she was her intimate partner. That was hidden by society all of these years.

One noon a black limousine pulled up and deposited Isak Dinesen and Marilyn Monroe and her husband, Arthur Miller, at the door of McCullers's white, three-story house. On her tour of the United States, Dinesen requested to meet only two people, this writer McCullers and this actress Monroe. The great Danish writer insisted on eating only three things, so this is what was served at lunch: white grapes, white wine, and white scallops.

I stand over McCullers's grave, her mother buried next to her, on a small hill, the river in the distance. I read her pink marble headstone that records her name and her two important dates: the month, the day, the year she was born and then her death in 1967 at age fifty. I think, *She was still alive when I read her in high school in 1964.*

"Thank you," I whisper in reverence. I place a small stone I find nearby on the top of her mound. I was here. I reach out across the years—across life and death—to say, "Your writing meant everything to me."

Edward Hopper's grave, whose childhood home is in Nyack, is nearby, but I do not search it out, though I very much admire his paintings. Not this time. I want nothing to dilute this singular visit.

4.

In late October of 2013, I traveled to Japan for a month on a trip with Upaya Zen Center. Joan Halifax, one of the leaders, arrived from India with a bad cold. I kept my distance from her and was proud that I managed to ward it off. I could not afford to get sick.

I arrived home late on a Sunday night, right before Thanksgiving, and slept in Monday morning. When I awoke and went into the kitchen, Frances, the cleaning woman who had worked for me for ten years, was sweeping. I went to greet her—then stopped dead in my tracks. She was coughing, clearly sick with the flu that stalks New Mexico when the season first turns cold.

I said from a distance, "Frances, go home. Don't worry about cleaning. You're sick."

She grabbed her coat and the check and slipped out the door.

Three days later I came down with the same flu. No way I could have avoided it. She had touched every inch of the kitchen.

The flu arrived in my body, and it would not leave. Three weeks turned into four, five, six. I struggled out of bed and then collapsed in a chair. The New Year came and went. I couldn't get better.

I asked for the name of a good oncologist from my primary care doctor and made an appointment.

For the second time I pulled open a door next to the word CANCER on the wall. Yu-kwan was beside me. She was living in Santa Fe now, in my old art studio, two miles from me. The flying back and forth became too much, and I think New Mexico, after thirty years in Manhattan, was an adventure for her. I often thought of the dust accumulating on her dark furniture in New York. The plan was for her to live half-time in Santa Fe, but she rarely returned to the city. She had no time— I had to show her the red hills of Abiquiú, the Jemez hot springs, the cows, the deer in fields. She had to taste green chiles rellenos, burritos, tacos—all New Mexican style—and how could she miss a sunset, the green of cottonwoods, or how the snow fell on piñons and junipers in the Sangre de Cristos.

The oncologist this time was lovely, warm, cheerful, and willing to answer any question. She told us that immune boosters can actually feed the cancer, which uses the booster to grow. You name it—echinacea, Ester-C, goldenseal, osha root, olive leaf, zinc, oregano, Chinese herbs, homeopathics. I had taken every one of them when I had the flu, the way my friends did, but had never understood why they didn't help me like they helped them. I only managed to spend a lot of money.

The doctor felt my neck, underarms, groin. No enlarged lymph nodes. I didn't have night sweats. This was good: no outward manifestation. The white blood cells were high, as usual, but nothing else too alarming. The oncologist said I must still be at zero. I mentioned I had irritable bowel syndrome.

"Maybe we should do a CAT scan," she said. "Find out if anything is inside that we can't see."

A week later I met with her alone. I felt sure nothing would show up on the scan results.

The oncologist, Dr. Rudolf, said, "The scan shows you have a ring of enlarged lymph nodes surrounding your abdominal aorta."

My cancer was lymphatic, and the lymph system spreads throughout the body. My cancer had a huge territory in which to manifest and park itself—in addition to traveling around in my blood.

"Why is the cancer there?" I asked.

"This is just a theory, but we think it attacks where it first began, the weakest point." I pictured all of those cookies in the café years ago. "I'm concerned that if the lymph nodes keep enlarging, they can cut off the blood flow to your legs."

"Am I still at zero?" I asked, holding tight to a past glory.

"I'd have to say you're now at one."

That's all I had to hear. "Who is the best oncologist in the country for CLL?" I asked.

She told me. "Dr. Irving Buckingham at MD Anderson." She added, "It's impossible to get an appointment."

"I'll get one." Alert, focused action was something I knew well.

The next morning I called everyone who had a remote connection to Houston, or to Texas, or to anyone in the medical world. *Think, Nat. Who do you know?* No one I contacted had a clear conduit to what I needed, but everyone said they would do what they could.

At three that afternoon the phone rang. It was Dr. Buckingham's receptionist. "Buckingham wants to see you at the end of next week."

"I'll be there." I still have no idea who got through.

• • •

Yu-kwan and I flew out. It was February, but in Texas it was warm, with soft air and small buds hinting on branches. A shuttle drove us from the hotel at 6:30 a.m. We wanted to walk, but MD Anderson was a city unto itself, and we would have gotten lost on our own.

Three other couples boarded the bus. They were

veterans, old hands at this early travel. I looked at them. It was clear with the Kansas couple who had cancer. The man had a thin, drawn face, a right hand that shook, downcast eyes. His head leaned back against the window. His wife attempted cheerfulness. "It's snowing now where we live," she said, meaning, *It's better here*. No, it isn't. She knew that. We all did.

The lights were stark in the hallways. Even the rickety elevator in the old part of the building was glaringly lit. I looked at Yu-kwan. She looked green in the light.

We entered the sprawling new section. It wasn't clear where to go.

Eventually we found the right desk. I was handed an iPad to fill out forms. I didn't own an iPad or an iPhone. I struggled to use the strange keyboard to answer simple questions such as name, address, and birth date. I punched two letters in, had to delete one. This pattern continued until Yu-kwan grabbed it from me. "I'll do it."

Yu-kwan was dressed up. She had done research on this number one doctor, Dr. Buckingham. She had watched videos of lectures by him and told me that we should be respectful around him. But I had not dressed up.

A gray-headed man around seventy walked through the lobby. Yu-kwan jumped up like she had just recognized Mick Jagger, "Dr. Buckingham!"

He was so startled by her enthusiasm that he grabbed her, and they locked in a big hug.

"Wait a minute. *I'm* the patient." I leaped up and also hugged him.

Then he backed away. "I'll see you soon," he said, and he disappeared behind one of ten thousand beige doors.

A few minutes later we were in his small office. He had a medical fellow working with him—a young doctor with an English accent who was there for advanced postgraduate training. Clearly, he also wanted to be connected with this star doctor. I mentally referred to this fellow as *the pipsqueak*. I had cancer; I had traveled all the way to Houston. I didn't want to meet with a nervous, inexperienced physician who clearly worshipped Buckingham and danced for his praise. But I allowed him to examine my body in front of his mentor to show off his knowledge, which seemed thin.

It was a fast exam. Then both doctors quickly pushed me to begin treatment with a new monoclonal antibody—a target therapy that aimed at the cancer cells directly, rather than taking down the entire immune system.

This involved twelve treatments—eight once a week in a row, then one treatment once a month for four months. "You'll go into remission for two years," they said, "and then you'll be ready for ibrutinib. It's our standard regime for the elderly."

"Wait a minute. I'm not vintage. I'm only sixty-six."

They explained that in the cancer world, anyone sixty-five or over is considered old and must be treated more tenderly. They said it's important to avoid chemo, if possible, because it knocks out the whole immune system. Then Dr. Buckingham said, "We want you to begin treatment immediately."

I shook my head. "I came here for a consultation, not to begin anything."

Dr. Buckingham looked stern. "We're afraid the ring of enlarged lymph nodes will close off your lower aorta."

The two of them played off each other. Pressure, fear, act quickly. No time to think.

Pipsqueak gave me a prescription for twenty prednisone tablets. "Begin tonight and you'll be ready for treatment tomorrow."

"I want to see what my blood results are first," I said. I was scheduled to go to a lab down the hall right after our meeting and get twenty tubes of blood drawn from my narrow veins.

Dr. Buckingham nodded. "Fair enough. But my recommendation stands. Let my office know what you decide."

After the blood work, I had to meet with five different social workers, clerks, and administrative assistants. We left the bowels of commotion and chaos in late afternoon.

That night in the hotel room, Yu-kwan researched this new treatment, the name of which was impossible to pronounce. It had a long list of possible serious side effects.

I was calm, talking intermittently to my Minnesota friend Carol, who was a physician, and who was also doing massive research into my cancer and Dr. Buckingham's proposed treatments.

The question was: Should I start tomorrow? In a month I had paperback editions of two books coming out. I also had a plan to meet with longtime students in Atlanta to sit at Martin Luther King's grave, and then go on an idiosyncratic tour of bookstore signings in North Carolina. A month after that I was going to France.

I gazed out the big hotel window, then flopped on the bed, staring at the ceiling, while the wheels of research at the nearby table and in the snows of the Midwest churned out information.

Dr. Buckingham had assured me I could quickly do four treatments, if I started right away, then wait until later, after all of my trips, to do the next four.

"Uh, Nat, I don't think you'll be robust after even one," Carol warned.

The next morning the pipsqueak met us in the office. "Where's Buckingham?" I growled. He scurried out like a squirrel and rejoined us when Buckingham made his entry.

They raised the pressure on us. *Better to begin here at Anderson, where we're experienced with this new treatment. The first time, you might have some complications that we can easily take care of.*

I called my oncologist in Santa Fe, "You'll be very

tired. It will be difficult for you to travel home right away." That made sense, but I finally gave in. I didn't want to be completely stupid. The fact of my cancer was now evident even to me.

I rushed upstairs to the pharmacy to fill the prednisone prescription. It was a Friday, the worst time to begin. If anything went wrong, only doctors on call for the weekend would be there.

Each treatment, if all went well, would take eight hours. It involved dripping a solution into a vein in my arm. I was going to begin in early afternoon. I could possibly be there until late in the evening.

Thirty people's prescriptions were ahead of mine. I sat in the waiting room, paging through *Woman's Day* and reading about nutritious quick-to-make meals for families. I called my friend Wendy in California, told her I was going ahead with the treatment. She offered encouraging words, but I could tell she was astonished by my sudden decision.

Yu-kwan joined me at the pharmacy. "Look at this flier the nurse just gave me. They should have given us this last night." She thrust a colored pamphlet in my face. The side effects were so much more blaring in this pamphlet than anything we'd seen on the Internet. Even possible death. Of course, the pharmaceutical companies had to cover themselves, mentioning every possibility, though the chances of their happening were minute.

"Let's get out of here," I said. Yu-kwan nodded agreement. We grabbed our coats and ran down the back stairway.

I called Wendy from the stairwell. "I'm not doing it. We're heading for the Rothko Chapel and Cy Twombly's exhibit. It's too beautiful a day."

"Do not separate a woman from her art," Wendy howled.

I had cancer; I had to meet it, but the threat of closing off the lower blood supply to my legs wasn't convincing enough right then. I also knew that cancer was counter-intuitive. Cancer cells lived outside human intuition. They barreled through the body and began to multiply, spread, and grow. Yes, in the future I would have to trust what the doctors said. But not this time.

Yu-kwan and I hit the streets like two escaping convicts. The natural light outside was calming. The last winter patches of gray and yellow grasses, the concrete curb, the changing red and green traffic lights, were a vision from heaven. I touched the bare branches. It felt as though they were about to break into blossom, though the buds were still hard stones.

I had visited the Rothko Chapel four years earlier. When I first saw the gray hollow of the chapel that Mark Rothko had designed right before he committed suicide, I could not relate to it. This time it resonated. It gave no consolation, no hope, no place to turn. This now felt honest, true.

The cancer would not leave me. What I had was a chronic condition. What I had was a human body that would die.

• • •

When I arrived home, I opened my computer to an e-mail from Nancy Conyers, a student who had studied with me intensely years ago. I'd heard she had breast cancer. She included a link to her essay "This Is What Cancer Does," which was published on *The Manifest-Station*. I opened and read the first paragraph:

> This is what cancer does: it makes your body unknown to you, an alien presence dragging 50lb weights on each ankle and around your neck. You are exhausted, so exhausted physically and mentally your brain can't send proper signals to get your unresponsive limbs moving. One time, for three days, you couldn't even wash your face because it was too much effort to lift your arms. When you couldn't stand your own smell anymore you tried to take a shower. It wasn't your own body odor you were smelling, it was the drugs you'd been infused with: TCHP, Taxotere, Carbo-platin, Herceptin, Perjeta. They were seeping through your skin, through every orifice and the metallic medicinal smell was making you as nauseous as the drugs were. You turned on the shower but the weight of the water pushed you against the shower wall and you struggled to turn the water off. You sat soaking

wet on the side of the bathtub until your spouse came to check on you.

My first thought: My, she has become a good writer. She expresses herself well.

My second thought: No thought. Blank. My heart screamed, *All this is not possible.*

5.

THREE MONTHS AFTER visiting Houston, in the middle of May, I met with the Santa Fe oncologist just before I was to leave to lead a writing retreat in central France. A lymph node on the right side of my neck stuck out. It was the first outward physical sign of my illness. She felt another swollen node lower on my neck. I ran my fingers over them both.

"I don't think I can let you go to Europe for a whole month," she told me.

After months of grinding avoidance and resistance, I surrendered. Just like that—I gave up. "Can we start tomorrow? If I wait over the weekend, I'll chicken out. I have to act right away."

I knew this meant canceling everything for the rest of the summer—not just the French retreat but the film conference, the Taos party, the weekend travel to Colorado to meet an old friend.

I went home and composed a letter to my students. They had all bought their overseas plane tickets months ago. I engaged two of my longtime students to take my place.

> With deepest regret, I won't be able to travel in June. But I want you to go anyway. I want you to swim and float in the lake for me, to see the sun rise over the green pastures, be in the old stone barn converted into our zendo, and sit in the circle, breathe with each other, hear the bell ring, share your writing, study even harder the assigned books, walk in the afternoon the trails and country roads to small farm hamlets past wildflowers and brown Limousin cow herds. Eat those French fries, baguettes, local cheese, that amazing butter, salade verte, everything from scratch that chef Thierry makes for us from food in a ten-mile radius and serves in that white stone dining room. Let nothing get in the way of your coming. This is about practice. You signed up. Be there to Sit, Walk, and Write. I will be there with you.

The students had to read *Madame Bovary*—it came alive in that rural setting—*The Belly of Paris* by Emile Zola, and *Paris France* by Gertrude Stein. On the last day, Dorotea, during formal tea, would surprise everyone by reading aloud the madeleine section of Proust while they all sipped local herbal tea and nibbled at those supreme cookies made in a local oven. My students would not go uncultured. But now they would go unteachered.

I was miserable. I'd looked forward to this for months. Everyone would be there but me.

After writing my sweet letter, I burst out crying.

Each day, after two infusions, shot up with that monoclonal antibody, the pharmaceutical name of which I still failed to pronounce correctly, I talked to the retreat, as promised, for an hour on Skype. What could I say to them, tanned and happy in another reality? I quoted Basho, the great Japanese writer, and asked them more about themselves.

It was June in my garden. The grama grass was growing long out the window as I talked across continents and the large ocean.

Buson, a lesser-known haiku writer, leaped into my mind and I recited:

> I go,
> you stay;
>> two autumns.

That haiku quivered through me. Death felt so close in that moment it broke down any defense. *Here I was. This was my life.*

Unplanned, I looked straight at that Skype screen, at my darling ragtag students on creaky chairs and *zafus* a million miles away and recited another haiku:

> On a single blade of grass
> a cool breeze
> lingers

I pronounced the haiku writer: Issa.

I put my hands together in a bow and snapped off the computer.

I turned my attention to what was in front of me. To what was in me: cancer. I finally met it.

• • •

Cancer doesn't hurt by itself; instead, it moves in on organs—the lymph system, the lungs, kidneys, intestines, even the tongue, and the brain—and cuts off vital functions. I liken it to mistletoe, suffocating and strangling the branches of the piñon in the mountains around my home. Nothing personal. The mistletoe wants to live—everything wants to live. Working in my garden, I watch this imperative to survive—the roses, the poppies, the raspberry plants, even the young cottonwood, twist over each other and over the fence to get sun.

Cancer cells come from the body. That's hard to contemplate. We think of cancer as a monster from another planet, but it's our planet, only slightly twisted, turned, reeling. In my case it was the white cells. They begin in the bone marrow, but the cancer cells don't fully develop, so they can't fight disease. They either fill the bloodstream or park in the lymph nodes.

We all have cancer cells, but usually our immune

systems recognize those cells and destroy them—or, as one oncologist explained, they are recycled through the spleen and are used again. Nothing wasted.

But with cancer, the body stops defending itself, can't recognize the cancer cells to stop them.

I meditated in the morning and spoke my thoughts to those alien cells. *Listen, you are young, not well developed. You don't know better, but it's time you leave. Do it of your own volition: This is a warning. A war will be waged against you. You'll be destroyed.* This was my gesture toward nonviolence, toward my friend John Dear, the Jesuit nonviolent activist. This was my gesture toward his work, a nod to King and Gandhi.

On another day I told them: *We've traveled together for a long time. It's time to go our separate ways. Adios.*

I did not feel hostile. My rage was against time. *Not now,* I said. *I am in the fullness of my life. I know at eighty I will still not like it, but for God's sake, leave me alone now.*

My acupuncturist said her Indian teacher often repeated: *You do not want to run neck and neck with cancer. You want to step in front of it and stop it in its tracks.* Meaning don't mess around trying herbs, potions, incantations. Cancer must be terminated.

I wanted my illness to be something simple, resolvable with the right homeopathic pills dissolved under my tongue. Or some spiritual, exotic problem. Too much dry heat in my liver or kidneys. Definitely curable by some kind of herbs. Something outside the realm of the medical profession, with its long hygienic halls, oppressive lights, and rigid appointments. My friendly attempt at relationship with cancer was absurd. Cancer cells won't leave on their own. Most every friend who had cancer and did only alternative medicine is now dead.

I had to enter the strange industrial cancer world. The big machines, the sterile rooms, the multimillion-dollar research. I knew I had to do this. I wanted to survive. I wanted my best chance.

6.

THE SECOND FLOOR of the Cancer Center in Santa Fe was lined with black lounge chairs and long cords attached to infusion pumps, which measured and administered drugs into patients' arms. Big windows all around provided a view of the Sangre de Cristo Mountains.

Every once in a while a bleep sounded or a light went on, alerting the nurse that someone's time was up. In my case the bleep was a signal to hang above my head another big, thick, clear plastic bag, like a cow's udder, full of medicine that it dripped infinitesimally slowly into a vein in my hand. I arrived at 8:00 a.m. I was the first patient each day. I was released at five o'clock, if all went well.

My friend Annie Lewis sat with me the first four hours every time. I met Annie in Ann Arbor in 1972, when we discovered we were dating the same man. In spite and rebellion, we leaped into our own uncensored love affair. Back then she was getting a PhD in anthropology on a full fellowship, and learning Hausa, an African language. The next summer she went to Santa Fe to attend anthropology film school and never returned to academia or the Midwest.

Sitting in the infusion room, we recalled how in Santa Fe she took evening acting classes. She reminded me as we sipped water (must stay hydrated, the nurse urged): "The teacher asked each student to stand up and speak *from your deep heart*. That's the four words she used. When I stood in front of the twelve other actors at the edge of the wooden stage, I threw my arms open and out ripped the statement: 'All I really want to do is sing rock 'n' roll.'"

"Where did that come from?" I jiggled the cord to the electric lounge chair I was lying in.

"I sang soprano in the choir in church as a young girl. Maybe that was it." Annie put together a band called the Quadrosexuals and was the lead singer, with blue hair, high heels, and a fitted one-piece leopard jumpsuit, her right shoulder bare.

When I moved to New Mexico a year after Annie did, I saw her on an outdoor stage with Allen Ginsberg, performing together. He croaked his Buddhist chants and she improvised lines in a cross between screaming and singing. "It was called *Sprechstimme*, a German word," she told me as a volunteer approached with a basket of chips, cookies, pretzels.

When the band fell apart, she and three other friends opened the Collective Fantasy, a small venue for foreign art films with a café attached. It was an anomaly in the seventies. She baked the brownies they sold. "Only with honey, not sugar. We were very idealistic."

"I can trace your life that far," I said. "How did you make the transition to bookkeeper?"

"After we sold it the new owners changed the name to the Jean Cocteau—by the way, do you know the theater finally landed in George R. R. Martin's hands?"

"I vaguely know the name." I stretched out my right arm. The catheter was in the left.

"He lived in Santa Fe, was a struggling writer, loved the Collective Fantasy's popcorn. Then he wrote *A Game of Thrones* and it all changed."

"Oh yeah, now I remember. He's a really nice man." I swiveled my neck around. So many hours to go.

"I needed something steady, sedentary, calculable, putting numbers in small boxes. I wanted off drugs. I was happy to gain weight and have some padding. I was too lean and on the edge of nerve."

"When people ask about you, I tell them that you were Phi Beta Kappa as an undergrad."

She threw back her head and laughed. Her hair was

now pale blond, short, and she wore baggy beige pants and a trim white, button-down shirt. "You're the only one it matters to."

We ate our lunch together. I had brought an egg salad sandwich and some chocolate sweetened by a god-awful sugar alternative that supposedly would not feed cancer.

After Annie left in the afternoon to go to work, my friend Susana arrived to keep me company for the second shift. She wore high-styled, understated French fashion, something gray and perfect.

I looked her up and down. She'd dressed up to visit.

Susana spoke fluent French and Spanish, was brought up in England, lived across the valley from me in an ancient adobe. I once visited her aging parents in Nice, France. Her father attributed his strong constitution to eating six apples a day and personally shopping daily for those apples. He died at ninety-nine. Her mother died at ninety-six. They had been married seventy-five years.

A volunteer asked if I needed another pillow. I shook my head no.

We talked about Susana's two one-woman plays. I went to each at least three times, taking in the humor, the poignancy, and the language.

She told me about the recent clothes she'd bought. I mostly do not notice what someone is wearing. I buy no clothes for a year at a time and dread entering a clothing store. I almost didn't believe Susana's interest in garments. After all, she read the *New York Times* thoroughly every day and was up on politics—not only America's but the world's. I often relied on her for updates and analysis. Even better, the girl read literature. Thick books did not intimidate her.

Now, with so many hours ahead of us, I had the space to accept the pairing of fashion and informed intelligence.

As the days passed and Susana spent one day after another with me, I leaned in to her interest in fashion. I said to her, "I remember it clearly, a Tuesday in January. It had just snowed when you and Stephen popped over to see my new house and studio. You were standing at the door to my studio, reaching for the knob when—don't you remember?—I noticed your new coat, the one Stephen bought you in France." The coat had a rough wool weave and some pale purple in it. "What amazed and delighted me," I told her, "was that I noticed it, woke up to a certain beauty I had been dead to."

In the infusion room with Susana I developed a curiosity about style. I showed her an elaborate ad for a turquoise purse in the *New Yorker* and a frenzied page for Ray-Ban sunglasses in *Rolling Stone*.

In that sterile cancer room, I quizzed Susana: *What is fashion? Why fashion?* I approached the subject as an anthropologist. I still wasn't interested in going any closer to the clothes racks, but as the weeks went by and we settled into our routine—Annie mornings, Susana in

the afternoons—I noticed everything Susana had on—
the turquoise sneakers, the black nylon pants.

During week seven of the infusions I convened a literary salon in the afternoon during Susana's watch. I had
been working on a rough draft of a new book. Susana
had just read it, and so had my ex-girlfriend, Michele,
who drove up from Albuquerque. Usually a discussion
with a friend about my recent writing lasted at most an
hour. But we had the leisure to fill the full afternoon
with discussion. After all, I wasn't going anyplace.

Susana liked the Zen essays at the end best. Michele
surprised me. She was partial to the hiking story. We discussed: *What is a book? What is story?* And the inevitable
question, *Who is the audience?* Near the end we fell into
a satisfied silence.

Michele left soon afterward. Susana and I watched
the last drops travel from the bag hanging over my head,
down the tubes, and into my veins.

The nurse, eager to go home—I was always the last
one to finish treatment—ripped the white tape off my
left hand and pulled out the needle. No matter how good
the discussion, as soon as the needle was out, Susana and
I bolted for the door.

We charged down the stairs to the ecstasy of outside,
even if it was just a paved parking lot. We jumped into
her bright yellow car and zoomed down the road, jolt-
ing over the speed humps too fast—anything to *get us
away from there*.

We skidded up to my front driveway. I grabbed her in a hug and then dashed out the passenger's side. Another session down, the aberrant cells tamed, I hoped. I was determined they would not run wild in this body.

· · ·

After each infusion I would open the front door and enter the kitchen. How the same, and how totally different, the stove, the refrigerator, the window over the sink looked. I was home, but I could not leave behind the memory of the infusion room, where all around me men and women entered, fell asleep, were discharged. All received chemo treatments, often delivered through a port in their chest. A man with dark eyes, olive complexion, a straight nose, so beautiful across the room it took my breath away. How could someone that beautiful have cancer? His wife sat facing him, bent over her large purse. They did not speak. They were done in an hour and a half. The next week he was much more sallow, yellow, thinner. He was dying, and everyone could see it. I watched a nurse, who had administered his drug two minutes earlier, sob behind the door so he couldn't see her.

7.

My dear friend Wendy flew in from California and accompanied me for my third infusion, giving Susana and Annie a small break. This was the second time I received two thousand units, the full blast.

After this treatment I lay in bed delirious with a high fever and bone-rattling, teeth-chattering chills. Wendy administered cool cloths to my forehead. For long hours she sat alone at my dining room table, writing her seasonal gardening column for *Tricycle* magazine:

I had planned to write this column on haiku and flower viewing. Forget that. The only flower garden I am getting close to these days is the antiseptic infusion suite of the cancer center. Here, "infuse" goes back to the Latin *infundere*, meaning to pour in, saturate, permeate, souse, and fill up for eight hours, once a week, the pale blue veins of my gutsy friend with 2,000 units of monoclonal antibodies.

The medicine my friend is receiving is relatively new, approved in 2009, with the mythic-sounding name of ofatumumab. I learned this a few hours into her treatment. It was quiet in the infusion suite, church quiet, resignation before the sermon. "The name of your meds sounds like Oh Fat Tuna Man," I whispered to my supine friend. She opened one eye, a wise and ancient sea turtle coming up to the radiant surface of the ocean, schools of tuna far below. We began to laugh, timorously at first, then raucously. Patients rose up in their recliners to stare at us with a mixture of amusement and horror. I noticed a little balcony off the main treatment room where we received immediate permission to relocate. Thunderclouds and the memory of rain saturated the landscape. We whipped out paper and pens. "Ten haiku. Go!" my friend commanded. Five-seven-five: Basho, here we come!

And so we split open piety and prudence that afternoon to receive a new infusion at the dark rim of medicine and disease. "Don't imitate me," Basho commanded his followers. "It's as boring as the two / halves of a melon." In response my friend recited her blunt verse:

> Rained last night
> Slow drip into my veins
> Sixty-six with cancer

We wrote and read to each other all afternoon. We ate brown rice and corn enchiladas and guzzled ginger kombucha. We reminisced about the battered green Chevy pickup under the cottonwood, and for long stretches of time we kept completely quiet. When the infusion was complete, I noticed with surprise that it felt like we had been gardening together. My friend told me then about Shiki, a modern haiku master who died of spinal tuberculosis at the age of 35. For Shiki, she said, the act of creation entailed alert stillness and infusion of intention. He dragged himself to the edge of his tatami mat to overlook the garden:

> One whole day
> Tilling the field
> In the same place
> *(translated by Peter Washington)*

After this treatment it became clear that a full dose was too much for my body. I spiked fevers of 105, alarming my doctors.

I took a week off from treatment. I had programmed myself: *Boom boom boom, let's get through it. Don't think. Just do it. 1-2-3.* But my body couldn't handle it.

My next treatment day was on a Friday. On Thursday I snuck off to the woods alone. I parked at the Chamisa trailhead. Two miles up and two miles down. I'd hiked this trail often in the past and thought it would be easy, as it always had been. But at every curve I had to stop; at every small incline I sat down. Under the ponderosas and piñons, the reality of how much my body had diminished soaked in. *I can't even climb Chamisa?*

Eventually, I made it to the top. I leaned against a tree, opened my notebook, sobbed and wrote, wrote and sobbed. It didn't matter what I was writing—it was all cause for tears. I probably wrote a continuous scream (I never reread it). But I came in direct contact with the groundless disaster—I could not hold on to my old life; I could not manage or form a new life.

I gave up on writing and decided I'd do *zazen*. Enough with words. A strong cross-legged posture, breath in and out, would save me.

I leaned against a straight-up ponderosa for support and crossed my legs.

I wept the full time. Not snivels and whimpers. Full-out squalling.

The shadows of trees passed slowly from right to left. I looked at my watch. Three hours had passed since I had gotten up there.

As I climbed down, my legs ached even more. I braced them against rocks, knees feeling the pull of gravity.

At the parking lot, my car was the only one left. Though it was the end of June, the air still had a chill as the sun went down.

How would I face the infusion? I did not under any circumstances—even to be with thoughtful Annie, faithful Susana—want to enter that infusion room, have them plug up my veins for eight hours, and be sick for days after.

But the next morning I was there at 8:00 a.m.—raw, subdued, pale. And we began again—but this time the prescription was reduced to a thousand units. I was told, and believed, that my body could bear it.

• • •

I found a balance with Oh Fat Tuna Man—with the one thousand units I was taking each week. No fevers, no chills. *Maybe this isn't too bad. By the end of October I'll be done. My blood work is excellent.* "No cancer can live with numbers like these," my oncologist repeated. My white cells are smack in the normal range for the first time in decades. *Okay, Nat—a year off and then I'll get back on the old horse and ride.* I have been *inconvenienced*, but it is temporary.

I watched my mind grab for reason, for time. Time was my only treasure chest. How much? In my mind I cornered off the year. Made my problem digestible, acceptable.

But I did notice, when friends visited, subtle differences. Yes, they had more energy, more mobility than I did. They were still busy in the world with the routines—the jobs, workouts, hikes, plans—they had before. No interruption. But there was something much more subtle, something I often didn't catch until after they left: *They don't know they will die*. It was constantly with me now, my mortality. It hung out on my right shoulder like an animal, patient yet hungry. It wanted me, and I knew that eventually it would have me.

I asked myself in the face of it: *How do I live?*

I recalled the Buddha's last words: *All things that are born must die. In any case continue with vigor.*

Meanwhile, cancer was proceeding for me.

HERE WAS MY
BELOVED'S LIFE

I'm in Missoula, Montana, a place I've been heading for ever since I read the poet Richard Hugo back in Minnesota in the early eighties. He lived, worked, and died in this town.

A few days earlier, I e-mailed Peggy Christian, a student who lives here. She studied with me a single week eight years ago. Peggy, who normally never reads astrology predictions in the local paper, saw this week's message: *An old friend from far away will be contacting you. Old Friend from Far Away* is the title of one of my books, published in 2008. When Peggy saw *from Natalie* as the subject on the e-mail, she thought a friend was joking with her. But I wasn't joking. I told her I'd need help navigating this town.

Hugo was known as a regionalist, and many of his poems are titled with the names of small broken towns in the Northwest. But what he writes about is not contained only in those places. He writes about death, other people's graves, loss, loneliness, land, drinking, how we bear up, how strong in the end we are.

Peggy and I visit the Missoula Cemetery. We run up and down the rows. No Richard Hugo. She calls a friend on her cell, then dictates directions to me. "A northside cemetery over the tracks on Cooley, Saint Mary's Cemetery, 641 Turner Street, flat marker under a huge elm tree." I jot down notes.

We stop at a small brick building, and I go out and talk to a nun. Peggy and I are now both mad to locate this grave. The nun confirms that Hugo is buried here.

We park the car and begin our search.

There are many big trees. Up and down we go. Up and down again—and a third time. She's at one end and I'm at the other. We yell to each other, the dead be damned.

Hugo wrote: *I don't want to admit / It's cold alone in the ground.* . . . I'm sure he wants to be found. *I say they put the dead / here where north and east gales can find them.* But we can't find him.

We finally give up, and she takes me to the Milltown Union Bar—a place where he spent a lot of time. He wrote a poem there that begins, *You were nothing / going in and now you kiss your hand.* We sit at the long bar and order beer. It's late afternoon. Peggy points out the elk head.

She tells me that when her mother died, she drove her mother's ashes in a box in the front seat of the car for four weeks to all the places her mother'd been and loved. She drove through Wyoming, Ghost Ranch, Taos—where her parents were married—Arizona, and finally up through western Colorado. She spread her mother's ashes in the wilderness meadow on the Flat Tops where her dad's ashes were spread twenty-five years earlier. She went home by way of Moab and the Canyonlands, her father's

favorite place on Earth. *What a wonderful way to grieve,*
I thought.

The day darkens. We didn't find Hugo's granite stone, his dates 1923–1982, and the words written there from one of his poems: *Believe you and I sing tiny / and wise and could if we had to / eat stone and go on.* But he's still here with us now, all over Missoula, not contained anywhere. I found him in our talk and drink and walking the rows and driving the roads with big sky over us and the Clark Fork River running through.

If I stay alive long enough, I'm coming back. I want to place my own small stone on the site where he's buried and complete the honoring of how much he means to me.

8.

CANCER WAS TEACHING me how to carve out and live in a small space. I had to narrow my vision to stay on top of the drugs, the appointments, the weird changes in my body. The world shrunk to what was in front of me, to my immediate needs. Zen all along was trying to teach me to pay attention: this single sip from this cup of green tea—green tea was supposed to be a cancer preventative. This button on my shirt—unbutton it, it's too hot. Even the screech of car brakes out the window—this, too. I'm still alive.

On a book I signed for a friend, I wrote the date. I did not take the date for granted. I got to live this hour, this day, week, month, this summer. How many more summers would I have? The night crickets, the late evening light. Sleeping with windows open, slam of the screen door, the ripening of green plums, the holiness of peach flesh, the thick shadow of trees full with leaves, my own skin exposed in short sleeves, capri pants, no socks.

Over the time of the infusions, I weakened. Too tired to go anyplace, I sat in the garden in a fading Adirondack chair an old friend from Minnesota bought me twenty-five years earlier. The cherries ripened on the tree in the corner. I did not jump up to weed, turn over the compost, tie up a protruding branch of a rose plant. Too spent to do anything, I listened to the aspen leaves tinkle in the breeze. I closed my eyes for a moment, taking in the sound. It was something familiar. My eyes jerked open. *I have cancer. I must be on guard.*

• • •

One afternoon in mid-June, Yu-kwan quietly lay down in bed and did a self-exam of her breasts. She had not had a mammogram in eight years. Without mentioning it, she made an appointment for a test.

She told me two days later on the phone, "I've felt a hard lump."

"Yu-kwan," I said, "you don't have cancer. *I have cancer.*" Maybe she was sick of caretaking and wanted some attention?

Wendy was still with me. When I got off the phone I turned to her. "Great. Now my girlfriend might have cancer." I kicked over a book on the low table. "Who's going to take care of me?" I was not on my best behavior.

"With all this cancer talk she probably got nervous that she might have it, but that's impossible." I opened my arms wide.

Yu-kwan's mammogram results were negative, but she told the attendant, "No, I feel a lump," so they automatically gave her an appointment for an ultrasound. She had to wait a week.

A week later, the radiologist told her, after looking at the ultrasound, "Cancer is on top of the list." She pointed out the rough edges of the mass.

Yu-kwan had to make an appointment for a biopsy and wait three days.

When Yu-kwan told me what the radiologist said, I was irate. "How dare she tell you ahead of time! She doesn't know! She should have let you have a few more days of peace."

I called Wendy, who was now back in California. "She might really have it. What am I going to do?" And I began to sob. I heard Wendy's sobs on the other end.

Yu-kwan got her biopsy on a Friday, then waited until Wednesday for the results. The waiting was the hardest part. I watched her pace the living room, even take out the garbage when it was only half-full. She sat down with a magazine, then popped up to open a window. My body was so drained all I could do was just watch. I'd never seen her like that. My heart ached, but still it was unimaginable—how could she also have it? And at the same time?

I did not go with her to any of the appointments. A friend offered or she went alone. Already we were separating out our cancer territories.

On Wednesday morning my friend Bill Addison, who came to see me from Atlanta, and I were in the kitchen when the phone rang. I ran to pick it up, calling to Bill over my shoulder. "It's probably Yu-kwan with the results."

"I have it. I have to find a surgeon. They're giving me info. I'll call you back later." And she hung up.

I placed the receiver in the stand. "Bill, she has it." I'd been dumped into freezing water. I couldn't move. My body was gooseflesh. I couldn't absorb, take in this information. *How can this be?*

Bill took us both out that night to the fanciest French restaurant in Santa Fe. He insisted on treating, though I knew his money was tight. I understood this was a sweet gesture in his need to do *something*, but I hated the restaurant. Every mouthful was rancid, sour, unappealing.

Bill, who is a food critic, thought it was good. So did Yu-kwan, who ordered escargots and calf's liver in onions. Nothing stopped that girl from eating. She also had a big dessert.

I thought they had no taste, that they'd gone crazy to like the food. I was sick with worry, stunned in horror. Yu-kwan was going to get a mastectomy and lose a breast?

I'd read about heads, arms, feet, hands, cut off for punishment. Now, right in front of me, it was about to happen. Yes, for a different purpose—to save a life—but the civilized world couldn't conjure up anything better? The world that could create bombs that turned corners, cars that could parallel park without the driver's assistance, could not do better than this approach to breast cancer?

Yu-kwan wanted to act fast. She traveled down to Albuquerque almost every third day, getting tests, meeting with oncologists.

A woman from the literacy board she was on—I'd never met her—stepped forward. She had recently had breast cancer and knew all the doctors, medicines, choices. She drove Yu-kwan down to Albuquerque regularly, waited for her, discussed her options, gave her books to read.

I was relieved. No way could I listen to another type of cancer's ins and outs.

Yu-kwan decided on a severe, young, precise surgeon at the University of New Mexico Medical Center. We didn't discuss her choices. She announced them. She would get a mastectomy, so she did not need radiation. There seemed to be no involvement of the lymph system, only that damn tumor, so she might even get away with no chemo.

She was hoping for a low oncotype score. For this score they analyze the genetic makeup of the tumor. *The tumor has its own genetics*. If the score was below 17, she wouldn't need chemo. If she had a score in the 20s, she should consider chemo. If the score was higher, she shouldn't take a chance. Yu-kwan was hoping for as little intrusion as possible. Losing a breast was enough.

Mostly I agreed with her, but I was also preoccupied with my own cancer.

We were aware that we were both on our own.

• • •

Yu-kwan, now retired for ten years, drew on the skills, power, and determination she had used to become an executive vice president on Wall Street for three decades. Starting in the late seventies, she was a woman of color when only men worked in those competitive information technology jobs and with those room-size computers. Even with her cancer, she was able to absorb enormous in-depth research. Whoever she talked to in the medical profession thought she was either a doctor or a scientist.

Logically, you'd think that we would commiserate, since we both had the cancer. But it wasn't like that. We each longed for caretaking, and neither of us had the energy to do anything but handle ourselves.

Any time we did try helping each other, we ended up fighting.

"You don't understand."

"No, *you* don't."

I did intervene one time. Yu-kwan's best friend, who used to be her girlfriend fifteen years earlier, was going to fly in for the surgery. I liked Nelsie a lot. I knew she and Yu-kwan talked often on the phone, sharing tips about day-trading. Yu-kwan once told me, "If Nelsie says buy, I sell. If Nelsie says sell, I buy."

The plan was for her to come for five days.

"Yu-kwan, that's not enough," I said. "Ask her to come for ten days."

"No. Nelsie has cats. She can't leave her cats." Yu-kwan paced the bedroom. "Besides, I can really do it on my own. No one needs to come."

I was lying in bed, watching her hands open and close in fists.

"Not long enough," I said. I knew it was hard for Yu-kwan to ask for help. "I'll call Nelsie myself."

To my amazement the little titan did not protest but walked across the room to get the phone and handed it to me.

The phone rang in the evening dark of the East Coast. "Nelsie, Yu-kwan needs you longer than five days."

Yu-kwan grabbed the receiver and heard Nelsie's response. "Okay, I'll figure it out."

"Can you?" Yu-kwan asked in her soft English accent.

When they hung up I said, "Feel better?"

She pursed her lips, which meant *I can still do it myself,* but then she added a nod. "Yes, thank you."

In nine days Yu-kwan's left breast will be removed. I counted down the days in my mind as mornings and afternoons passed. Then my brain would stop. The air felt thick, ponderous. It felt as though we were carrying heavy sacks on our backs and had trouble moving toward each other. Time itself became awkward.

"Should I try to come down for the surgery?" I asked one morning.

"No, your infusion is right before. Even though you're handling it now, you're so weak."

"I'm sorry," I said. "I can come afterward."

She shook her head. Yu-kwan was not being tough right then. More resigned. Nothing would help.

Everything was moving so slow—and so fast. Any energy we had was poured into practicalities: "What will you bring? A toothbrush, toothpaste? I hope you can get out after one night. Do you want to bring some food with you? Those almond butter packs?"

"I don't think I'll be hungry." She attempted a small smile.

I reached out my hand and ran it along her arm. I leaned over and kissed her, but it had such a different resonance than it did before. Instead of passion, I could hear way in the distance the low sound of a bell tolling.

Two nights before the surgery I asked again, "Are you sure I shouldn't come?"

"No, didn't Ann say she'd drive you down the next day? But only if you feel up for it—and only for an hour. Who knows if I'll even be awake."

Nelsie did come for ten days, flying in the night before the surgery. They stayed in an airport hotel to be at Yu-kwan's 7:00 a.m. appointment the next day.

Days later I asked Yu-kwan if she slept that night. "I had to. We were getting up at five a.m." They went to bed at nine.

I thought for the thousandth time, *That girl can sleep*. Even when she was getting a breast removed the next day.

I lay in bed all morning, exhausted by the recent eight-hour infusion of Oh Fat Tuna Man, waiting for Nelsie's call that it was over, imagining my dear girlfriend's beautiful breast being removed.

The call came. Nelsie said it went well, whatever that meant in this situation. Then she handed the phone to Yu-kwan, who was sobbing uncontrollably. She had girded herself to take care of all the details, determined to rid herself of the tumor, to do what was necessary. Now she was in shock.

She was also drugged. She'd leave the hospital the next day. "Don't come," she told me.

My good friend Ann came over anyway, and we sat in the red chairs in the living room having a rich time writing together. How was that possible? Partly because I was in my own drug and cancer daze. Also, both Yu-kwan and I developed a fierce selfishness during that time. We grabbed any small pleasure we could get.

I said to Ann, "Do you think this is okay?"

"Better than stress and worry," she assured me.

Ann was right, but still it haunted me. How far had I gone from normal human reactions? I'd been taught we weren't allowed to be okay while someone we loved was suffering. I don't know what rule book this was written in, but certainly in my childhood, chaos and hysteria were the proper responses to distress.

I called Wendy to tell her the surgery was over. "Wendy, have I become dead, evil, comatose?"

"No, Nat, you are out of it. You and Yu-kwan are smart. If it were Peter, I would have crawled on my belly along the highway to get there. Who would that have helped?"

Nelsie dropped off Yu-kwan at my house when she left the hospital, then went off to pick up groceries and fill a pain prescription, which Yu-kwan refused to take.

"All I need is some Tylenol," she said.

Standing in the front doorway, she looked old and defeated. Her posture was askew, her left shoulder leaning far to the right from the lost balance that two breasts provide.

I helped her off with her black coat. As I slung it in the closet, I sensed a hug was out of the question—her whole chest was bandaged.

I took her by the wrist and led her to one of the red chairs in the living room. "Tea? A cookie?"

She shook her head.

"I know, how about if I run a bath?"

"No bath!" she screamed.

Of course, the raw wound—what was I thinking? I swung my head around and looked at her again. I hid a gasp and hoped I covered the horror I felt.

• • •

A week later her onco score came in. She was hoping for 20 or less. Instead the score was in the 50s—so high even the doctors couldn't believe it. They sent it back to be redone. The second score returned. Still in the 50s.

She had been lucky. She noticed the cancer early, before any lymph node involvement, but it was growing fast. It was over an inch in size when it was removed. She needed chemo.

Not only her breast—now she'd lose her straight, pageboy-length black hair too.

9.

I WAS IN LOVE with Yu-kwan's loveliness. Her small ankles in the short gray socks with the gorillas at the anklebones. Her black Spanish shoes with heels clicking across my cement floor. The perfect narrowing below the calf. The pout of her thick lips. The graceful arch of her neck. Her shoulder bones jutting out of a thin sweater.

We rarely argued. Whenever I carried on about how she needed to exercise more, make friends more, eat less sugar, she simply responded, "Yes, dear." It oddly satisfied me, the older, bossy sister in my family, as though I were only searching for an agreement—the hell with what she actually did.

Occasionally, I'd snap my head around and say, "You're not listening to me."

"No, dear," came right back. The absurdity stopped time and we both giggled.

Here I was, an American, grandchild of Eastern European immigrants, in love with an Asian woman. For the last forty years I'd been studying Eastern mind, dedicated to Zen practice. But Yu-kwan, an immigrant herself from Hong Kong via England, had no innate interest in Buddhism. She delighted in the opportunities America afforded her. She felt an eagerness and care for her new country, just like my grandmother did—enthusiasm, imbued with hope for a better future.

Our first meeting was simple. Yu-kwan was the partner of a writing student I had fifteen years ago. Because they both worked full-time, when I taught a weekend writing retreat in New York, my student insisted Yu-kwan come along.

I'd heard about Yu-kwan in earlier retreats Alice had attended. She wrote about the commitment ceremony they planned, the bowls of roses, the designer dresses. She told me at lunch about her new girlfriend's beauty. I was happy for Alice and half-curious.

The New York retreat had eighty students, most of whom I'd never met before. As I walked from the back of the room, Alice waved her hand, and a small Asian woman stood beside her. *She's not that pretty*, I thought to myself.

Yu-kwan was quiet in class, but she grinned a lot, and when she did, her face lit up. She wrote a ten-minute timed writing about being a pig—eating too much. This surprised her, her first attempt at creative writing—and she was delighted, beamed throughout the morning.

I surmised she understood deeply what I was teaching, with its Asian roots.

During a break, I went over to her. "Tell me, what do you do for a living?"

"IT" she whispered.

"What?"

She repeated the initials.

I must have grimaced—something to do with technology?—and walked away. Back then I didn't even own a computer.

Many years later, one August afternoon I ran into her in Taos. She'd broken up four years earlier with Alice and had come to say a final good-bye to the town where Alice had had a second home and where they often vacationed.

Walking with a friend down Kit Carson Road, I saw her in the distance, standing in front of a gallery. "I have a vague feeling she's someone I know," I said to my friend, pointing. As we came closer and I saw her face, I knew I knew her but couldn't place her.

"Hi," she said, that big grin, her white teeth.

"Hi," I said back.

She could tell I was computing in my mind. "I'm Yukwan. Remember? New York? Alice?"

"Ohh," I said, then jumped in. "Yes! I even remember

during a break I ran into the two of you in that old café near the class. I had just ordered chocolate ice cream. The walls were green. . . ."

"Yes, yes," she said excitedly.

An unusual cloud moved overhead, oblong like a train, and I pointed. All three of us bent our heads back.

Yu-kwan glanced at her watch. "I've got to run. I have a massage. Great to see you." She rushed off, and I watched her cross the street at the light.

I turned to my friend. "Maybe I should go out with *her*?" I'd just been lamenting no dates for a long time.

We e-mailed for six months, my long missives responded to mostly with two or three lines and then an occasional long e-mail telling me of her day. It might have gone along like this for even longer, but as winter approached, she invited me to New York for my birthday to see *Turandot* by Puccini at the Met. It was an opera about a ruthless, cold Chinese princess softened by love.

But first she would fly out in late December to go snowshoeing and see a movie about Paris that, amazingly, wasn't showing in all of New York. She wouldn't let me pick her up at the airport. Instead I met her at the shuttle in front of the Hotel Santa Fe.

The night was cold and dark, and she popped out of the van in a heavy green coat. I handed her a dozen pink tea roses, and we went to an Italian café near the Plaza, where the food we ordered went almost untouched— we were nervous and absorbed in each other.

Intermittently she patted her lips with a white cloth napkin, and I thought I had gotten it all wrong. She was the most beautiful woman I had ever seen, and her beauty emanated from the inside out. She glowed.

In New York she presented me with an expensive pen. A terrible gift choice. I only use fast-writing cheap pens and spiral notebooks. This Rebecca Moss pen was slow and too thick. Hadn't she read any of my books?

We bumped along seeing each other. Once in Texas; she'd never been in that state before. I had work there, and she came early for the weekend. I gave a keynote in Washington, DC, and she met me there. We walked under the cherry blossoms along the Potomac, and I told her about Japan and my love of Japanese authors. Eventually she bought my one-bedroom studio in Santa Fe, where she had sometimes stayed in the past, so we could date properly—in the same town.

Slowly, the recognition of her true, sweet, odd nature unfolded inside me. I noticed she told the same joke over and over. When a restaurant meal was brought to the table, she would say to me, "What are *you* eating?," meaning she was going to devour everything we'd ordered together. I never failed to laugh.

She never walked barefoot, even in the middle of the night to use the bathroom. She'd grope for her slippers before her feet landed on the floor. I asked, "Is this a Chinese thing?" in my vast ignorance, and she shook her head no, with no further explanation.

For her birthday I worked hard on a painting of a homemade coconut birthday cake. To the left of the cake was an old-fashioned mixer and mixing bowl; a chocolate chip cookie was prominent on a plate to the front right. All on a checkered tablecloth with rose-flowered wallpaper in the background. I was afraid I might have overworked the layers of color, trying too hard to get it right.

I presented it to her the morning of her birthday. She glanced down at it on the table in my studio, then walked over to the house, saying nothing. I thought, *She hates it.* I decided not to ask.

Two hours later, she looked up from the newspaper as she turned the page, "That is the most wonderful present anyone has ever given me."

I grew to love and be fascinated by her long silences.

And her huge generosity. For Valentine's Day she surprised me with a large red oil painting I'd admired in a gallery a month before, and then a small oil as the Valentine card.

On the first night I spent in her New York apartment— on the ninth floor, lulled by an old memory of the soft hum of traffic below—I slept for twelve hours straight. That single night of long sleep sealed the relationship.

The silk of her legs, and the depth of her ability to relax, awakened longing—I could learn this ease from her, this unrestricted acceptance, and recline into peace.

But that tranquillity was still foreign to me. On a hike two weeks later, back in New Mexico with my friend Erica, who was also my local doctor, I tried to explain this quality of deep relaxation.

"Nat, she's a cat," Erica said as we huffed up a challenging mountain. "The rest of us are dogs, eager to be petted, acknowledged." Erica made short panting sounds. "Love me, love me." She hung her tongue out.

"Yes, yes, that's it," I laughed.

On a bench outside, a few months later, Yu-kwan began for no reason: "This is how cats lick themselves," and she extended her lower arm across her tongue and then the other arm. She turned her head to the left and raised her upper left arm, nuzzled and licked under her armpit. "This is how they get clean."

My eyes twirled in my head. She looked exactly like a feline. "Did you ever have a cat?" I asked.

"No, never."

"Then how do you know?"

"I just know."

That night, when I couldn't sleep, I listened to her breath, heavy, then slightly snoring, then snoring deeply, then silent, never using a pillow. In a pale yellow nightgown, she was out in space, against aging and time, arms outstretched over the whole dark world.

Later, feeling the fragrant heat of her breath, I shook her awake. "Sing to me," I said, and she obliged, still hovering someplace else. Out came a sweet rendition of the Beatles's "When I'm Sixty-Four." At that time we were both in our sixties, out beyond our generation's imagining, out in the footprints of the comets.

• • •

When Yu-kwan first moved to New Mexico, a year and a half after we began dating, I told her, "You have to learn to drive. We have no subway lines, and few cabs." I spread out my arms. "This is the West, big country," and then I added, "I'm not going to be your chauffer."

First, she stuck up her nose. "I can drive."

"Yeah, a license you got thirty years ago and never used."

"Watch me." The next day she went by cab to the Honda dealer out on Cerrillos Road and bought a tan Honda CR-V. From then on, for ten months the talk was of speed limits, traffic lights, left-turn lanes, parallel parking.

When she was at the wheel, I sat in the back seat, catching up on past issues of the *New Yorker*. I didn't dare glance up. Often I'd hear a car horn.

"That person is so rude," she said.

"You cut him off."

"I did no such thing. I had my directional on. I signaled."

"But you also have to look."

She snapped on the radio to an oldie station, singing along. "Stop! In the name of love"—she had a beautiful voice with a classical English accent.

Whenever my car needed a tune-up, oil change, or tire rotation, she gladly volunteered to take it in and always made a 7:00 a.m. appointment. (I thought, *That's efficient—in and out.*)

One afternoon she was upset. "I couldn't get scheduled till ten this time. All the good donuts were taken by then."

"They give them for free?" I was putting two and two together.

"Yes." She nodded. "No chocolates left. I had to eat one with blue icing and another with pink." She paused, smiled at the memory. "But they were good too."

"I thought you took the car to help me out and also to further your auto understanding."

"That too." A big grin spread across her face. "Last time, what do you call them? They had crullers. Delicious."

10.

I WATCHED YU-KWAN not resist being tired. Instead she accepted it and lay down on the bed or long couch in the back room, staring out the window at the aspens.

Our acupuncturist encouraged us to buy a lamb shank and drink the broth. "It's so good to build strength," she said. I did it once or twice, didn't like the taste, was bothered by the smell in the kitchen.

Yu-kwan persisted, bringing home that raw shank every other day, plopping it in the pot and waiting while it boiled. She poured a cup for herself and one for me. "C'mon, I insist you drink it."

"Why don't you drink mine too?" I sipped at it, making the ordeal longer than necessary.

She watched me quietly, a resignation in the way

she leaned over the sink holding herself up. "Do what's right. We have to do what is good for us."

• • •

Yu-kwan's mother fled China when the rest of her family was killed in one of the many empty revolutions Mao stirred up. Her mother gave birth to Yu-kwan at the age of seventeen in Hong Kong. There was no father nor a mention of a father. When her mother first met her stepfather, Yu-kwan was farmed out to a poor family at age seven for two years. Her mother was afraid the English soldier wouldn't want her if she had a child.

Yu-kwan's adopted family ate one bowl of rice a day and some salted fish. When they sat at the table, they kept their feet raised on the chair rungs. Rats came out at dinner and wandered under the table, hoping a crumb or morsel would be dropped. Barefoot, thin as a wire, she wandered the streets. The ghetto people called her "the wooden beauty" because she was so sad.

After her mother couldn't get pregnant in England, she confessed to her new husband that she had a little girl left in Hong Kong. Her husband flew back and appeared at the door of the boarding house. Yu-kwan was standing in the hall when the owner opened the door to this tall white Westerner. He told her to call him Daddy and yelled at the man that her mother sent monthly checks for her care, yet she was filthy and starving.

The next day he took her to the movies to see *One*

Hundred and One Dalmatians. She sat next to him with one fist full of popcorn and the other gripping chocolate malted milk balls.

For a short time, maybe six months—Yu-kwan can't recall the exact amount of time—the three of them stayed in Hong Kong. She said those months were the best time of her young life. Each Saturday, while her parents played mahjong with the neighbors, Yu-kwan slipped out of the house and took the double-decker bus—front seat, top deck—all the way to the other end of Kowloon. The ride took a half hour, and then she'd walk to the cinema. She had a favorite actor who played in the Chinese operas—she followed him by photos in the newspaper—and she'd sit in front of the screen, watching a similar plot unfold each week. He was always the hero, starting out poor but eventually winning the kingdom and the girl. If an English feature played nearby, she might go to it too—first the Pathé news, followed by a cartoon, and then a slapstick starring the Three Stooges. "You didn't need to understand the English; they were just funny."

On the way home—again front seat, top deck—she'd get off at her street. As the bus turned around at the corner, she'd race it to the end of the block with her long skinny legs. She always made sure to beat it, because then she would reward herself with a gateau at the bakery. It was a game she played with herself. Then she'd visit the candy shop, where she'd spend the last of her pocket money on one stick of Wrigley's chewing gum and a single sweet-and-sour hard candy.

At home her parents were still playing mahjong. No one looked up when she came in the door or asked where she'd been all day.

This was after the Second World War. Soon the family moved to Germany, where her stepfather was transferred. They sent Yu-kwan to an English boarding school. They changed her name to Violet, thinking that would help her adapt more easily. She became Violet Jones.

"It sounds like a porn star," I told her.

English was the first language she learned to read. The kids bullied her and made fun of her for being Chinese—"Violet" didn't help—but this was where she learned the power of her own essential nature. Her mother told her, "Fight back."

Her mother had a cobbler make her very first pair of shoes when she went off to school. They were made to last—too large for her, she'd grow into them, with metal around the edges. She hated them—another reason to be made fun of. She even stuck them under the tire of a parked car, hoping they'd be crushed when the car moved. It didn't work—nothing could destroy them—so she turned those shoes into a powerful weapon.

She calculated her moves. She waited for each bully to be alone, and then she'd use those shoes to attack.

The big, overweight, fleshy leader of the bullies was her most ambitious target of revenge. One day, at the edge of the school campus, Yu-kwan saw her walking on the sidewalk. She ran behind her, and with her sturdy shoe, kicked her hard in the butt. The bully fell over, her thick glasses flung out of reach. Facedown on the concrete, she stretched her right arm out for them. Yu-kwan rushed ahead and was about to crush them with her huge shoe.

"This is where you develop who you are, your character," she told me. "In a split moment I changed my mind. I reached down, handed her her glasses, said I was sorry in English, and walked away."

"She bounded after me, gave me three of her marbles, took my arm, and pulled me to the playground." From then on they were best friends, the skinny short Chinese girl and the big white Brit.

Because of Yu-kwan's great effort to learn, her sharp ability in math, and her appealing face, her teachers took a liking to her and kept her close. She learned perfect hygiene and elegant manners.

The English kids were well fed. Her early childhood had been marked with hunger. She developed a zest for kippers, baked beans, roast beef, and Yorkshire pudding.

Her mother stopped her from drinking milk. "You'll grow too tall and won't find a Chinese husband."

Half of Yu-kwan had no idea she was Chinese, because the language in which she first learned to read and do equations was English. Her first ten years in Hong Kong were amorphous, bent on survival and the exigencies of chance. But learning to decipher words, building the obtuse logic of numbers, even sitting in rows in a class-room—the dailiness of repetition began to form her character with a British lilt.

She developed a highbrow accent, as if she and Queen Elizabeth frequently had tea together. Her Chinese voice was lost in her clear, precise pronunciation of this new language—syllables and consonants at attention, her strange way of pronouncing *aluminum, schedule, vitamin,* like swimming in a dark and separate sea. Though she often dropped articles of speech: "I go to bathroom."

In her sophomore year of high school, one spring afternoon she beat the 100-meter women's world running record by two seconds. The physical education teacher went crazy.

The dean called her parents, who decided that her stepfather would work to train her all summer. They purchased new running shoes and shorts and sleeveless cotton T-shirts for her.

The first day, alone with her stepfather on the deserted summer field with so much skin exposed, she felt vulnerable, unsafe. As she'd grown into puberty, he had begun to notice her in uncomfortable ways, and one rainy afternoon a year earlier in the hallway to her parent's bedroom, he'd reached out and squeezed her left breast. *This running practice is going to go on every day for two months?* she thought.

She walked off the track, telling him, "I don't want to run anymore." No beseeching changed it.

Her mother never really learned the new language, became more isolated, insecure. She beat Yu-kwan with a stick. "Why aren't you nicer to your stepfather? He loves you."

"My stepfather used to take me to the movies. One afternoon we saw *Peyton Place*. In the movie, the stepfather impregnates his daughter. I watched and a light went on. *This could happen to me.* I was certain my mother wouldn't care if I became pregnant by my stepfather. It would be one way to keep him. She'd raise the child as her own.

"That day I began to plan my escape. The neighbor woman used to hear my shrieks as my mother hit me. Twice she called the police."

"What happened when they came?" I asked.

"My stepfather was in the army. He talked to them. They wouldn't go against him."

When she was eighteen, her neighbor drove her to a distant airport. She'd saved the ticket money to fly to southern England. She had a friend there with an apartment she could share. She packed very few things and snuck her passport from the top drawer in her parents' bureau.

She never saw them again and was alone, with no aunts, cousins, uncles, brothers, or sisters, no kin at all.

Her aloneness became her family. It stayed close, and she knew it thoroughly, right to the ground.

When I met her, her mother and stepfather had faded into her past.

"Don't you want to know if they're still alive? Where they are?" A true American, I could not leave it alone, thinking everything can be changed, made better, have a happy ending.

Surprised even at the question, she said, "No. Why would I want to know? My mother hated me. And also abandoned me for two years when I was seven."

"But, but," I stammered, years of psychology at my back, "your mother was unhappy. She lost her family in China. She—"

"No." She cut me off and shook her head.

In one sense, Yu-kwan was the most mature person I ever met. She didn't expect her mother to be different, to fulfill an ideal image of mothering. She was able to burn through the pain and desire, and see the truth of her mother before her. Not expecting it to be other than it was. *This is the hand you were dealt; now sally forth.* Yu-kwan peered directly into the horror, the vulnerability, the luck or jinx of her life.

In the 1960s, at age twenty, living alone in London, she discovered Shakespeare's plays in the cinema. She thought, *Ahh, here's someone who understands me.* She dreamed of someday becoming a Shakespearean scholar.

Instead, living at the YMCA, with no money and no way to make a living, she wept when she was rejected by the secretarial school. "I couldn't type fast enough."

In the evenings an older woman resident at the Y taught her to play chess. Pretty soon she was beating her teacher.

"You're smart," the woman said. "You should go into programming."

"What's that?"

She took a six-month course, eventually taking a test that landed her in New York at Automatic Data Processing, where the boss was a legend on Wall Street. He wore long-sleeved white Oxford shirts to cover the tattooed numbers along his wrist—his identity in Auschwitz.

This New York Jewish company, which employed many Hassids, took Yu-kwan in, guided her through stocks and bonds and computers that occupied entire rooms. She eventually drafted the theoretical programs that other programmers made happen. The company hired John Lennon's lawyer to get her a green card.

My beloved became an Upper West Side New Yorker.

At age fifty-eight she retired. She did finally study Shakespeare, putting herself through four years of a BA at Sarah Lawrence. All the other students in her classes were nearly forty years her junior.

In the Shakespeare class, when it was her turn to recite a memorized passage, she chose *Othello*. She told me that, as she spoke the lines, *When you shall these unlucky deeds relate, speak of me as I am; nothing extenuate, nor set down aught in malice: then must you speak of one that lov'd not wisely, but too well*, tears rolled down her cheeks. She had a whole lifetime to know the truth of that great playwright's words. The students, in their twenties in desks around her, mostly theater majors fulfilling a course requirement, stared at her.

One called out, "Wow, you really feel this, don't you?"

• • •

It took me years to coax small details of Yu-kwan's past out of her. She didn't want people to feel sorry for her—or even worse, for them to feel sad, listening to her story.

One day she said to me, "I will tell you one thing, but you must never tell anyone." Then she fell silent.

My imagination went wild in her long moment of hesitation. *She killed someone. She has another lover.*

"What? What?"

"I had to take a GED exam," she whispered. "I never graduated high school."

"That's the big secret?"

"My stepfather came to visit the boarding school in my senior year. There was a used condom in the parking lot. He freaked when he saw it and pulled me out of school. He was very possessive."

"Didn't you protest when he took you out of school?" I asked.

"No use. All my childhood I was dragged one place or another, with no consent." She shrugged her shoulders.

"Yeah, but you found a power against him when you said no to running. Did you miss it?"

For a second time she shrugged. "It was a terrible choice I had to make, a self-inflicted internal wound. That day I realized I'd lost passion for things, and almost immediately I started losing time running when I went back to school. I no longer broke records. There was a psychological shift."

• • •

Now Yu-kwan had cancer too, her left breast removed. For the first time I saw her worry about blood relatives. In bed at night she divulged her fear. "Who will care for me when I can't take care of myself, when I really become helpless?" Each day she feverishly washed the dishes in the sink. "We can at least keep the place orderly."

She looked often in the mirror, anticipating clumps of hair falling out once her chemo treatments began. "I should get ahead of the game and shave my whole head now."

She called Jean, a longtime Zen priest, who was used to shaving a neophyte's head. "Would you do it for me, please? I guess I am undergoing some kind of transformation—but not a religious one."

"I'd be honored to help," Jean said.

On a Sunday in mid-September, the last of the tomatoes hanging on the vine and the peach tree leaves just beginning to turn, Yu-kwan sat in my back garden as Jean first cut Yu-kwan's black hair as close as possible with a scissors. Then, with shaving cream and a bowl of warm water nearby, she shaved my sweetheart's head with a single blade, working slowly and carefully.

"Wow, you have a beautifully shaped skull. You'd make a good priest."

When they were done, they dropped her long hair and the shavings into the compost bin. "Let the worms at it," Yu-kwan said.

Friends brought caps they'd knitted in anticipation of her bald head. Red, green, black, yellow, orange. She even wore them to bed.

"I feel like I'm sleeping with a schoolmarm," I told her.

"You know, it's cold without your hair."

She bought a wig but never wore it. One night I asked her to put it on for a few moments. "I want to try to remember what you used to look like."

She obliged. A black coif appeared on her head. She pranced around the bedroom. "Here I am." She flung open her arms—and then flung off the wig. "And here I really am."

DOWN TO THE MARROW

In 1986, the second time I go to Paris, I search out Simone de Beauvoir's grave. She is buried with her partner of fifty years, Jean-Paul Sartre, at Montparnasse Cemetery.

Graves are lined close to each other; no space for grass—every inch filled in, a whole cement city. When I enter, I approach a small man in a beige overcoat. I half-finish my inquiry in terrible French when his arm juts straight out, pointing in the direction of Division 20.

I want to make sure. "De Beauvoir?"

He nods and walks away before I can call out, "Merci."

I've already gone to Les Deux Magots, where Sartre and de Beauvoir met. There I poured hot chocolate out of a porcelain pitcher, nibbled at a crusty croissant. Here, in the Saint-Germain-de-Prés area of this romantic city, was where the two talked, devised philosophy, and shared the gossip of their liaisons.

The two were always linked, but it is Simone I want to visit in her cramped grave. To thank her for a single line in *The Second Sex* that I read in my midtwenties. It rang in my head like a bell, tolling the direction to my future. I paraphrase: *In order to create, one must be deeply rooted in society.* After reading that line I vowed to elbow my way in, to be heard. I knew women had been pushed to the margins.

Here she is below all of this marble, granite, concrete. I stand a long time. There is no loose stone nearby that I could use to mark my visit. I take an American penny out of my wallet and place it below her name.

Our lives pass. A link past death carried in her words.

11.

By September I was finished with the eight weekly infusions. Now I had four months of respite ahead with once-a-month infusions. What a relief.

I also had a two-week retreat scheduled in France for the end of September. All summer I had my fingers crossed that I wouldn't have to cancel that too. The oncologist said I could go. Yes, I was a little weak, but let me out of here.

A longtime student from Mexico flew into Santa Fe to escort me onto the plane. At each airport exchange a wheelchair took me to the next gate.

We hit the bright morning in Paris and rented a black car, drove down to Ferme de Villefavard, formerly a farm of one of my student's grandmother's, now an arts center.

I stayed on the third floor of a grand old dilapidated stone farmhouse, climbing three long flights of stairs. I insisted on this room, where I'd stayed before, with the two large dormer windows opening to the brown Limousin cows grazing in the long green grass.

Two days later I faced thirty-five students from England, Holland, Germany, Australia, and the United States. To my delight, at least ten women of color attended. Thirty years ago I'd had to coax a single Latino or African American or Filipino to join us. Times had changed. Thank God.

After an explanation of procedures and safety by the director, it was my turn to speak. I sat quiet for a long moment. The students might have thought I was searching inside for something profound. The truth was, at that moment I had nothing to teach. My mind was like the inside of a Ping-Pong ball. I'd taught for many years. I was sure I could pull out something—*Ah, writing practice!*— but no. It was all far away, in another land, before cancer.

Nat, say something, anything. "You have traveled from very far." Another long wordless moment. "You have pens. That's good." I looked around. "Ah, notebooks too." *Remember, Nat, you're a writer. The pen goes on the page.* "You know what to do."

And out they swam, far into their own minds and notebooks.

For those two weeks, I mostly treaded in thin thoughts, not daring to plunge.

One woman from Germany, who had a PhD from Yale, leaned in with a face of consternation—wrinkled brow, lips pressed together—whenever I spoke.

"Peggy, you make me self-conscious," I finally said.

"I want to understand."

"Don't think too much or the real grain of writing will never come."

She explained that every sibling in her California family of ten children had made it—lawyers, doctors, teachers. The older ones pushed the younger ones through. "But now," she told me, "many of them are paying the price. Alcohol, antidepressants, divorce."

Ah, the American way. "Write about that." She seemed to relax. She could write the truth.

As I crawled through the first week, I slept well every night, but in the morning I was exhausted, could barely move. Then I noticed my mouth was always dry and no amount of water quenched my thirst. And I was terribly constipated, which I credited to all the baguettes I was eating. I'm usually gluten-free, but in France the wheat is processed differently. I took advantage. Cheese and bread, bread and cheese.

The truth was, I was fading. But I had a retreat to lead—and lead I did. In the evenings I took fifteen students at a time on slow walks down the narrow country roads, listening in silence before the sound that rows of mature corn make in a light breeze, and watching fat lambs munch and jump in fields. We walked under sycamores, seeing pigs near wood shacks, and past rows of flowers along the edges of barns.

• • •

While I was in France, Yu-kwan had her first chemo treatment. Her stepdaughter from the previous nine-year relationship with Alice flew in for a week to support her. The first treatment didn't seem to be too bad, she told me by phone. But she was warned that the effects were cumulative.

How could I leave her to go to France? We had talked about it and came up with the simultaneous conclusion: *Go!*

"You're ready to bolt, to feel autonomous again," she said. "You'd be impossible if you stayed here. No help at all. The hope of France is what kept you going all summer."

"Are you sure? Am I uncaring?" I asked.

"I need you out of the way. Besides, I'd love to spend time with my stepdaughter. We'd trip over you." She leaned close. "I'm so glad you're up for it. Remember our vow: we each have to do what we have to do."

I called her each day, hearing my voice echo in the empty farmhouse hallway. Several times I couldn't get through at all, and I'd scream into the receiver, "Fuck you!" I'm sure my students heard me. "Yu-kwan, are you all right?" Only electric noise. It was a graph of the psychic distance we each created to survive.

• • •

I made it through the two weeks. But when I came home I couldn't get out of bed, and I had a constant cough. The kitchen seemed far away from the bedroom. I could not traverse the distance.

During that first week home, I had a blood test. My oncologist called the next day. "I know why you are so tired. Your calcium is very high. You better come in tomorrow."

Annie came with me. Yu-kwan, slowed down from chemo, sat at home by the phone, waiting for our call.

The oncologist told me, "Your cancer is active."

"But how? I thought I was okay."

"That cough. It could have spread to your lungs."

• • •

Yu-kwan watched me drag myself to the bathroom and listened to my panicked phone calls to try to get advice, appointments. Every clinic had a waiting list. I could see someone in a month. "Not fast enough. I'm full of cancer."

Yu-kwan continued to clean the kitchen frantically, scrubbing the stove top for the third time. I hung up, walked over to her, and took the sponge from her hand. "Enough." I pointed to the couch.

We didn't talk very much then. We were in our parallel hells.

Both of us had been on our own from an early age. Yes, I had parents, a sister, people I could call aunts, uncles, cousins—but I always felt desperately alone. I left for college at eighteen and never returned. I saw my parents once a year, but there was little connection or support. People would ask, "What do they think of your books?" They never read them. There were no books in our home.

I was a silent child who received little attention. But the silence I often had with Yu-kwan was different, comforting. I felt free to live in my own thoughts, wander in my imagination, relax deeply in the quiet safety that this other human being provided and accepted. For me it was a living Zen: to just be. Not nagged or criticized or having to constantly protect myself. This silence served us well. It allowed me the full screaming journey inside, the best way I knew to stay close to my own hard experience.

In our bones we both shared the deep loneliness.

• • •

I went for a CT scan and then spoke with my oncologist about the results. They weren't good. "I called Dr. Kind (yes, that was his name), a urologist, who said he'd fit you in for a consultation. You have an enlarged lymph node by your left kidney. I also have a call in to the doctor at MD Anderson. We have to get your calcium down. It's dangerous."

The next day I waited in a windowless room to see the urologist. A person in blue scrubs walked in. He looked like a kid in junior high. I wanted to point and say, "The soccer field is that way," but he sat down opposite me and began explaining that I had to get a stent placed in my urinary tract as soon as possible. He flipped through a chart. "I have a surgery opening for tomorrow."

"Tomorrow? Why? I thought this was just a consultation."

He rolled a machine forward that showed me photos and x-rays of the problem. He told me I could lose a kidney if we didn't do this soon.

"What about another day?" I asked. "I need a little time."

He adjusted his glasses. "I could also do Friday, but you need to decide soon. The spaces fill fast."

When I arrived home, there was a message from the oncologist. She'd heard from MD Anderson. An enormous amount of prednisone, administered through my veins two days in a row, should lower my calcium.

I called back and said, "No. That amount would make me psychotic."

She told me she would come up with a different prescription—but something had to be done.

Slowly a picture was beginning to emerge: those last four months of dripping Oh Fat Tuna Man into my arm had given the cancer a boost, free time to keep growing. All along it hadn't been working.

Looking only at the blood results each week hadn't been enough. The oncologist repeated, "With scores like this, the cancer can't exist."

Well, guess again.

The cancer cells this time were not in the blood but parked in my lymph nodes. And those parked cells, undetected, were having a free-for-all, a heyday. The high calcium was from the cancer eating at my bones and dumping the results into my blood.

The CT scan also showed that the enlarged lymph nodes circling my abdominal aorta had not gotten bigger but hadn't shrunk at all.

The oncologist called a second time. Even though I was coughing, I did not have lung cancer. But what did I have? The original blood tests showed CLL, but maybe I had two kinds of cancer, one of them that didn't respond to Oh Fat. I needed a biopsy of that lymph node circle. She gave me the number to make an appointment.

I hung up and sat in a chair, staring out the window. The aspens were brilliant yellow up in the ski valley, and from town they showed as patches of mountain gold. *We should drive up there.*

I convinced Yu-kwan to make the drive. I sat in the passenger seat. A long line of cars also wanting to view the autumn aspens moved slowly, then faster.

As we drove, I stared into my lap. I knew I couldn't stay with the comfortable, warm Cancer Center in Santa Fe, where over the months I had learned the names of all the nurses. Veronica, a single mom with two children in school, who was able to hit my vein right on the first jab. Kathy, my first attendant nurse, pregnant eight months with her second child, who assured me

I didn't need a port. Lorraine, raised in Santa Fe, who was having her wedding in Hawaii so all of her relatives wouldn't come. The Cancer Center was near home, three miles away.

I had made phone calls to the Mayo Clinic in Minnesota; to a different branch in Phoenix; to a blood expert in Seattle; to a student's brother-in-law, who was a cancer researcher in Detroit; to a connection at the NIH in Washington, DC; and to the University of New Mexico Cancer Center in Albuquerque. All of my life I had fastidiously stayed away from the medical profession. Now my life depended on it.

I trusted acupuncture, homeopathy, naturopathy. These made sense to me, but cancer made no sense. I was out of my league. I had to drop all of my opinions, my likes and dislikes, and fiercely go into the belly of the beast, the white-coated medical world.

As Yu-kwan concentrated on driving, I was deep in thought. *I'll end this life. I don't want to go on. I don't care about these autumn leaves.*

We arrived at Aspen Vista, enchanted people weaving among parked cars and motorcycles, heads tilted back, looking at the leaves against the blue, blue sky. We parked. I didn't move.

"Aren't you getting out?"

I shook my head. "I want to go home."

Yu-kwan's face jerked toward me. Without a word she turned the car around.

The whole drive back, I considered how to kill myself. I'd never been suicidal before. But the task of ending my life was practical and urgent.

An hour later, at home in the embrace of my sofa, I snapped out of that desire. I can't say how, but in the release of that hunger I remembered what a friend told me as we traveled by bus in Japan. He said, "One of the forms of craving the Buddha identifies is the craving for nonexistence." I had just been slammed into the truth of that teaching.

12.

I WOKE AT 6:30 a.m. with a need to get out of the house. I put on clothes and walked out the door. I had no energy. I walked the pace of a snail, the sun still behind a mountain, the light bleak. One foot after the other down the Cerro Gordo dirt road.

After twenty minutes I passed Upaya Zen Center, normally less than a five-minute walk away. I heard the wooden *han* calling students for *zazen*.

I went a little farther to a farmhouse. I knew the German owners were away. A little bit more and then I couldn't go farther. I stopped, sat down right there on the side of the dirt road.

A white car slowed. "Hey, Natalie. I saw you earlier, always practicing. Doing slow walking?" He was so cheerful.

I looked up, could barely raise the corners of my lips. "Yeah."

The white car rolled away and accelerated. Dust rose from its wheels.

Zen practice is for people with energy. Not for the soon-to-be corpses, I thought.

I glanced at the road. Was I seeing right? A bull snake, six feet long, fat in the middle, pale yellow with large spots, was making its way across. I knew these snakes. Once, when I lived up on the mesa in Taos, I found one curled on my *zafu* in midafternoon when I opened the zendo door adjacent to my studio. In a panic I called my friend Sean, who drove his rickety van over the potholed road to my place. Like a snake charmer, he let it wind itself over his extended arms. Then he carried it out into the sage. From Sean I learned that bull snakes were big but harmless.

Cerro Gordo was not a busy road, and at that hour few cars passed, but it would take only one to bounce over that snake to kill it. I was too tired to get up. I crawled into the road and lay parallel to the snake, six inches away. They'd have to kill me first.

Up close, I could see the snake had whiskers on either side of its nose. "C'mon baby," I whispered into the desolate air, the desolate day, this desolate life. "Move, keep going." Its face crawled past me into the dried, prickly ragweed at the edge of the road. Its long gracious body followed. I wound my way up to standing and walked home.

• • •

I scheduled the biopsy of the abdominal lymph node ring for Wednesday and the stent surgery for Friday. Every day that week I was stabbed for blood samples, until my veins gave out and it became harder and harder to find one. I'd never been so black-and-blue.

I showed up for the biopsy naive to how involved it was. The interventional radiologist had to put a needle deep in my abdomen, bypassing and not piercing any organ or intestine, and remove a sample of that swollen ring of lymph system.

A jolly nurse prepped me, and I was rolled from one waiting area to another. The surgical room was in use and not available. She kept assuring me everything would be fine.

I'd like to say all of those years of meditation kicked in and I was tranquil. That didn't happen. But I wasn't nervous either. I moved into a dead state of quiet and calm. I surrendered my animal body, like a prey animal when it knows it's caught. No escape. My body was no longer mine. I'd given up. *Take me.*

Only the area where the doctor was going in was anesthetized; otherwise, I was awake. He had decided his best shot was through my back. I lay on my side, facing away. I could not move. He had told me I had to stay stone still. No problem. I was already frozen.

Only when it was over and I turned around did I realize how dangerous a procedure it was. The doctor, using the back of his hand to wipe away the sweat running down his face, said, "That was tough. I didn't know if we could do it." Relieved and elated, he held up the sample in a jar.

The next day, Thursday, waiting for Friday's stent surgery, I was back at the Cancer Center with another needle in my arm. I was being hydrated. High calcium in the blood dries a person out. This drip was a quick Band-Aid. This time I was only in the infusion room for an hour.

We had to figure out something soon. I needed some kind of prednisone fix until we could decide how to stop the cancer.

Friday morning, when I showed up for surgery, my blood pressure had not gone up at all. My numbness had its advantage. I would get through. Sometimes that by itself is a victory. To get through. To continue to live.

I was wheeled into the freezing surgical theater with eight people in attendance. I saw the urologist, in a corner breathing deeply, bending at the knees, raising his arms over his head. He was warming up, getting ready. That stent had to go through my urethra up into my left kidney. As with an athlete, it took concentration and presence. I smiled under the ten thousand fluorescent lights. A needle was jabbed into a narrow vein. I went out.

I woke in recovery. Dr. Kind, touching my leg, "It went well. Your urethra was very narrow. I had to push hard."

But having the stent inside was miserable. Sometimes it hurt so much I could barely walk. But the alternative was to take it out and chance losing a kidney.

I kept it in. It would come out when we figured out how to get rid of the cancer. And so far no cures were in sight.

The following week I began a protocol of five tablets of dexamethasone, four milligrams each, per day. This would bring the calcium down to normal—and me to abnormal. The plan was that I would do this for four days, take a four-day break, and begin again. This was the compromise my oncologist devised, instead of the blast that the MD Anderson expert suggested.

In the days after I stopped taking the first round of the drug, all of my physical and emotional ailments were exaggerated, amped to forty times worse than they already were. Past hurts stepped forward as though no time had passed. Bitterness poured into every part of me. Twisted old defenses and armor reappeared. I thought I was going mad, with no place to land.

I managed to articulate my despair to a friend. "Maybe," she said, "it's about coming down from the drugs?" That had never dawned on me; I had been so lost in the pain. I grabbed that thread of reality—and slowly, as three more days passed, I lowered myself back down to the ground.

• • •

My last visit to the Cancer Center was oddly bittersweet. I knew I would be leaving—I needed a radical change to save myself. My oncologist in Santa Fe was a cancer generalist; I needed a specialist in blood diseases—a hematologist. I would miss this strange place and community I was thrust into. I knew the woman who made appointments, knew where the bathrooms were, knew the temp nurse who seemed to be playing a nurse in a sitcom but had no real idea what to do. I'd bark orders to her: *The bag is empty; time for the real stuff; the pillow for my arm is over there.* She'd smile, ignore me, and pop off on her way.

I'd miss the attendant who weighed me, took my temperature and blood pressure, and cheerily asked, "Having a good day?" I'd say things like, "This is a cancer center. I have cancer. Do me a favor, don't ask again." And each week she'd ask anyway and I'd roll my eyes.

I was there for another hydrating session; she saw my desperation and asked, "Stress level? One to ten?"

"Do you have an eleven?"

She took things into her own hands. She surreptitiously closed the door of the windowless room and as the pressure machine pumped my arm, under the brightest fluorescent lights in America, she commanded, "Let's pray."

Sure, what the hell.

We squinched our eyes shut and called on Yahweh, Vishnu, Buddha, Zeus, Aphrodite, Allah, the Holy Ghost, and whatever god trees came from in a thick one-minute vigil that rocked the calendar with the photo of a waterfall off the wall.

I would miss them all.

13.

ALBUQUERQUE, the biggest city in New Mexico, is like entering another America to people who live in Taos and Santa Fe. To get there, you drive south through the Rio Grande Gorge and down through dry pueblo land on I-25 at seventy-five miles an hour. From Santa Fe it's a straight sixty-minute shot to the airport. That's pretty much our relationship with Albuquerque.

When it rains in Albuquerque, it snows in Santa Fe, the mountain town that makes its living on art and tourism. Albuquerque has industry, jobs, and a new top-of-the-line cancer center. Now I had another reason to go south, to drop two thousand feet in elevation.

My first impression of the place: too slick, too institutional, too shiny and organized.

I felt claustrophobic, defiant. But the oncologist I met

with was efficient, quirky, and smart. Clearly, she knew her stuff. She suggested bendamustine and rituximab to treat the CLL.

I knew about bendamustine. It had been used in East Germany for thirty years but had only come to the States recently. It had very good results. I knew of an eighty-year-old in Santa Cruz who went into remission taking it.

But I also knew about the dark side of the drug. "Do you know Mark Keltz?" I asked her. Mark was an old hippie friend from Taos. A year ago he had a single treatment of bendamustine in this very place—for CLL, the same cancer I had. His bone marrow production was wiped out. Normally with chemo drugs, the entire immune system gets knocked back, but it returns within a day or two, or at least in time for another treatment. His didn't come back; for the past year he'd needed weekly transfusions.

"Everyone at the center knows Mark. It was a very unusual case."

"Well, if that happens to me on this stuff, it's over. I can't handle a year of transfusions."

"Then it's clear you should take ibrutinib instead."

Bingo. That was the drug I'd wanted from the beginning, back when I'd first heard about it in Houston. But it had just come out, and the FDA allowed its use only after something else—for me it was the fearsome monoclonal antibody—had been tried and failed. I wasn't eligible then because I hadn't yet tried Oh Fat Tuna Man, but I was now.

You took three capsules every day, and it didn't mess with your DNA or wipe out your immune system. It targeted B-cell malignancies, stopped the enzyme Bruton's tyrosine kinase, which is essential for cancer survival. The catch: you have to keep taking it as maintenance after the cancer is gone. I would never be drug-free. And ibrutinib had been out only a year, so no one knew how long it would work.

Cancer was insidious. I'd heard that sometimes, when a certain type of cancer is being destroyed by a drug, the cancer will morph into another kind that the cure doesn't treat. I think: *Only cockroaches and cancer will survive the atom bomb.*

"Ibrutinib is probably a better choice for an elderly person," the oncologist added after my long silence.

"Are you calling me old?" I'd already had a similar discussion in Houston.

This oncologist was knowledgeable and alert—but I could tell that if I became emotional in any way, she'd respond with statistics, facts.

I liked her, but she wasn't quite right. At the same time, I knew I couldn't be too picky. I had to begin some protocol soon. Back to square one: How do I find a doctor that's right?

I'd given up on going all over the country to find the

right doctor. I was too weak, and the stent was killing me. I needed treatment here in New Mexico.

The University of New Mexico Cancer Center had a growing reputation, and a family physician I knew in Santa Fe almost whispered to me, as though it were sinful ever to try to challenge the mighty empire of cancer in Houston, "It's as good as MD Anderson."

I called my former girlfriend Michele, who was a lawyer for the university. "Can you get me the name of a good blood doctor at the university?" I knew they were called hematologists, but there was pleasure in making them sound like Dracula—or curanderos.

She called me the next day. "I've got the name of a hemotologist who had to appear for a hearing. Everyone gave up on her patient as good as dead, but this doctor persevered and saved his life. My colleague said she knew her stuff." Michele hesitated. "He said she was a saint. Brought up in Albuquerque, only went to New Mexico schools."

"What's her name?"

"Dulcinea Aragon."

I called Dr. Aragon's office, but she was impossible to get an appointment with. I got off the phone and paced. *Who do you know? Who do you know?* I was back at zero. I didn't know anyone. *Think, Nat, think outside the box.*

A light came on. Rob Strell, an old boyfriend from when we were in our early twenties. We moved to New

Mexico together. Now he was a prominent designer and architect in Albuquerque.

I called him and left a message explaining my situation. "Do you know anyone who can get me an appointment with Dr. Aragon?"

Twenty minutes later the phone rang. It was Rob. "I know a child oncologist at the university who's best friends with her. His boyfriend has worked for me. He's sending you his e-mail and the information he needs. He'll give it to her tonight. She lives nearby."

Even then it took ten days to get an appointment with Dr. Aragon.

This oncologist had to be the right one. I couldn't mess around anymore. The cancer was gaining momentum, and the calcium wouldn't stay down long. So far that kick of drugs had squelched it, but I simply wouldn't take the second four-day round. It was only a matter of time before the cancer would gnaw at my bones again and dump calcium into my blood.

14.

Almost every evening, Upaya Zen Center dropped off food for me. Joan Halifax either called or visited every day. Whenever Rob Wilder cooked chicken, beans, and rice, he made enough for me and Yu-kwan. A woman I never met named Jane left elaborate macrobiotic food in paper containers at the front door. Susan Voorhees, my yoga teacher, cooked dinner for me every Tuesday. David and Mark down the road came around 8.00 p.m. on Thursdays with more chicken, chips, guacamole. The first time, they delivered brownies that David had just baked, still warm. I didn't tell him we had stopped eating sugar. I danced around the brownies for half an hour, then plunged in. One friend, who is not a good cook, hired a caterer to bring twelve frozen packages of chicken soup to be popped in a pot whenever we were hungry. I asked Susana to make her wonderful meatballs, and I ate them for days. Ann brought over a roasted chicken she cooked on a Saturday; Annie, gazpacho; Onde, chicken soup, nongluten breads. Yu-kwan came over almost every night for dinner.

The food was endless. Sometimes I wasn't well enough to eat anything, but something was always left at my front door— a woven basket full of fresh apricots, tulips, a mum bush, presents from my students.

Visitors I hadn't seen in the last six months were nervous when I opened the door. *What would she look like? A Holocaust survivor?* I'd lost twelve pounds, but I could afford it. In fact, the weight loss—and even more, all the rest, the not traveling, the being home all the time— was good for me. People's faces relaxed when they first looked at me. "You look good."

"It's the cancer, the secret beauty cure." What else could I say? *I may look okay, but I'm in hell.*

One friend, when I told her I'd canceled my June travel plans, said, "Oh, you'll get to see your roses."

I'd planted rosebushes helter-skelter when I first moved in and figured I'd made a mess of my garden. With the dry, hot weather we had in June, I was certain the roses would look terrible, but my friend was right. I was finally home enough to behold the pinks and yellows and reds. I had a real rose garden. It was gorgeous.

Some days I was way too tired to do anything, but I'd still walk outside and put my fingers in the soil. The flowers lived and died; the sour cherries, peaches, pears, came after white blossoms. The fruits not picked fell to the ground. No fuss. No complaints. They lived out their lives.

Each day the sun came over the mountains. Each night the coyotes shrieked. I loved this life. All of it.

• • •

The man who escorted me, Yu-kwan, and Annie to a small room to await Dr. Aragon told me, "She could work anywhere, but she has committed herself to twelve years here." His eyes filled with tears. He was proud of the homegirl.

Yu-kwan was still in the middle of chemo treatments. She wore the red woolen hat my friend Ann had knitted for her. This was the only time during her cancer that she came with me. She wanted to meet this doctor.

After a twenty-five-minute wait, which is short for these institutions, Dr. Aragon sauntered in. She wore a snappy black-and-white dress with nylons and heels. Young, probably in her thirties, pretty, with a big smile. She shook hands with each of us and sat on a stool opposite me. She asked us to call her Dulcinea, not Dr. Aragon. She explained that she had already consulted with the other oncologist. "We both agree—ibrutinib seems the best course."

I nodded. "Let's get it started." I already liked her, and I couldn't waste time.

"I have to write a prescription, and the pharmacist

downstairs will order it. They'll send it to your house. It shouldn't be long."

"And I just start taking it? That's it?" *Like an antibiotic for an infection? All my effort, machinations, now reduced to a dose a day popped in my mouth?*

"Yes."

• • •

Days passed and the drug didn't arrive. I called the pharmacist. She discovered that more paperwork needed to be completed first. "Where does your income come from now? You only get social security?"

I was desperate to start. "I have some savings. Please, maybe I could pay for the first month?"

"No, it doesn't work like that. And you don't have drug insurance?"

"I will, beginning in January. I got bad insurance advice last year. I might have a royalty check in November for a book I wrote." I knew it wouldn't be much, but I was embarrassed at this point to have no income.

"A what?" She negated that. It was too out of the ordinary for her. "I'll see what we can work out."

• • •

The phone rang three days before my next oncology appointment. "Hi, Natalie." I could hear it was Dulcinea.

"The ibrutinib hasn't come yet," I said.

"It's good you didn't start it. Dr. Smith and I presented your case to the hematology panel that meets once a month. They're so smart. We're so lucky to have them here. They are not convinced that you have CLL. Yes, the biopsy you got in Santa Fe says it is, but how do we know about other places in your body? They suggest you get a PET scan. That will tell us exactly where the cancer is and to what extent. From that map we can take several biopsies."

I blanched. "Several?"

"I agree, it's too much. How about if, after the scan, we decide then? They are concerned you also have lymphoma."

What kind of lymphoma? A PET scan? The appointment for the scan couldn't even be made in the radiation department, but in the *nuclear* department.

The test would be on November 4, a Tuesday. All of this digging around was postponing treatment.

• • •

Susana picked me up on the fourth at 6:30 a.m. She was not a morning person, but a tenderness I'd never seen in her before came tumbling out. It was still dark as we barreled down the highway. The sun peeked over the wide horizon as we hit Santo Domingo Pueblo, then San Felipe and its big casino sign. The Sandia Mountains appeared as we got closer to the city. I asked Susana to relay the international news she had read in the *Times* over her morning toast and cheese. None of it was good.

The receptionist at the scanning center was peppy, but I couldn't get her to fax the results to my doctor

Erica in Santa Fe. Instead, I would have to fill out forms and take them to another department.

She told us the scan would take two hours. She said to Susana, "Go have coffee across the way." She pointed out the door.

The room where I sat in a cotton gown was cold. The nurse couldn't find a vein to inject an intravenous contrast. Too much blood had been taken in the last weeks. My veins had collapsed. After three stabs I asked, "Please, can someone else try?"

She went to the emergency techs. A new person appeared. After two stabs, the needle went in. After a half hour of the contrast filling my veins, I was ready for the big white tubular machine.

The tech asked, "What kind of music do you want?"

"Classical, please."

She placed big earphones over my ears.

Intermittently, when she wasn't giving instructions, I could hear music, but over the *kick*, *bolt*, *crank* of the machinery, Mozart sounded like a cracked plate dropped over and over.

Eventually the scan was finished. I exploded into the waiting room.

Susana greeted me. "I was getting worried. It's been three hours."

"Let's get out of here." By now we'd become good at bolting.

Neither of us had eaten for hours. We got a restaurant

suggestion downstairs from a clerk near the exit. "Down Twelfth Street, in a residential area."

The corner café was already phasing over to the midday meal, but they let us order huevos rancheros, the special that morning. The frijoles were pale and bland, but it was enjoyable to try a new place in the foreign territory of this sprawling city.

I had noticed a sign at the front door: TWENTY PERCENT OFF ALL SPECIALS. I reminded the waitress when she gave us the bill, and she reduced the amount.

I smiled, knowing Susana, who was shy and proper, was aghast. They let us have breakfast when lunch was being served; that should have been enough. But I was a New Yorker and loved to flaunt my chutzpah in front of her.

· · ·

The very next day, Wednesday, November 5, I was heading down to Albuquerque again at a more decent hour: 9:30 a.m. Annie was a cautious driver, and we putted along in what felt like slow motion. I was in no rush to hear the PET scan results.

Dulcinea walked in and handed me the report. Annie was poised with her notebook and pen to jot down comments. ". . . Hypermetabolic activity is present throughout thoracolumbar spine, ribs, sternum, scapulae, and pelvis, suspicious for high-grade involvement. . . . Lymph nodes: markedly hypermetabolic . . ."

At this point I was retreating down some barren highway in Nebraska, a long time ago, in another life.

I came back for a moment to hear that my marrow was rocking out with cancer. "Activity throughout, markedly avid nodes above and below the diaphragm . . ."

Now I was back on the highway. *I think I'll stop at the next Conoco, get me a Clark bar. Do they still sell them?*

"We need to get a bone marrow sample. See here." Dulcinea showed us the lit areas in moving pictures on her computer. No way around it—the cancer was ablaze, "Most of these areas are technically difficult to biopsy, especially adjacent to vascular structures." She paused and shifted over to a diagram. "But here, where we normally take marrow samples through the hip bone, it's also lit up, so we can do this safely."

They were going to drill through my hip bone. I finally spoke up. "Okay, we have to do it right now. Not tomorrow, not late afternoon. I can't think about it. Right now."

She got it. "There is a lot of cancer," she said again, and then ran out of the room to set up the biopsy.

Twenty minutes later I was lying on my right hip. A very competent nurse was numbing the left hip, where she would go in with a needle. Her words were reassuring. I relaxed and made conversation with the assistant, a homeboy, as the needle plunged through my skin, my muscle, my bone. "Tell me some good places to eat here in your hood."

He named some, all Mexican.

"Any other kind?"

"Nope, never go to anything else."

"Indian? Italian? Chinese?"

He shook his head.

The nurse said, "We're almost there," meaning the needle was reaching down through the bone into the marrow.

A minute later I felt the needle withdraw. "I've got it. You can turn your head and look."

I saw a jar of liquid. Floating on the bottom was what looked like a mushroom section with gills exposed.

"Some people are sore after. Some aren't. The results will be here on Friday or Monday. Dr. Aragon will call you," The nurse said.

Ten minutes later, patched up, I met Annie in the lobby.

I didn't want to drive home right away, so we went to Bookworks on Rio Grande Boulevard. A few stores down was a dress shop. I limped over to it, my hip very sore. I bought a gray cashmere sweater for myself and a bright cardigan for Yu-kwan's birthday the next week.

Annie and I hardly talked on the drive home. It was dark out and I'd dawdled as long as I could before returning to Santa Fe.

Yu-kwan swung the door open. "You're so late. Where were you? What are the results?"

We were standing in the hallway. Annie hesitated,

then started to tell her, withdrawing the results from the folder.

I listened for about a minute, then exploded in a small tantrum. "I'm going to bed." I dropped my purse and coat on the floor, ran into the bedroom, and slammed the door.

As I lay in bed, I heard their voices through the wall, intense and undecipherable.

I had been battered for the last six weeks—needles, tests, biopsies, drips, machines, sterile waiting rooms, stiff chairs, long waits on the phone filled with Muzak. It had been nonstop. *Think, Nat, think. What can you do?*

Once before—more than a decade ago—I was on a weeklong Zen retreat in Saint Paul. On the sixth evening, when I went home to my small third-floor apartment, vulnerable and open, I made the mistake of picking up my mail in the lobby on the way upstairs and opening a letter from an old acquaintance. I read something that set me off in waves of anger.

That night in bed, I tossed and turned, infuriated. *Nat, all of this sitting and look at you. Stop.* But I couldn't.

Then, right in the middle of this struggle with anger, I fell below all the turmoil into a place of complete peace and open space. All of my muscles relaxed.

This state continued through the night, and the whole last day of practice, until we bowed out in late evening.

During that afternoon I had a formal one-to-one

meeting with the teacher and told him what happened. "That peace is available all the time," he said.

"But how did I get there? It was like I fell through a hole." I felt buoyant, underwater.

He shrugged his shoulders. "Sometimes when you struggle like that, something comes up to meet you."

Something similar happened to me that night in bed in Santa Fe, but this time I understood it. Underneath everything, I was struggling to survive, to stay alive. I simply let go, simply stopped struggling. Whatever was in the bone marrow, it was already there in my body. Nothing I could do but let the drama unfold.

• • •

On Friday, when the call did not come, I was relieved. I could relax through the weekend. *Enjoy this time*, I repeated to myself. The song we learned in high school French class, which turned out to be an American song written for Doris Day, *"Que Sera Sera," whatever will be, will be*, whirled in my head.

On Monday morning at ten, Dulcinea called. To my great surprise—I'd already let the worst happen—the marrow showed it was still CLL. "Start the ibrutinib pills."

"They still haven't come," I said.

The next day they arrived via Fed Ex. I signed for them, and the red-haired woman standing at my front door handed over a small white box. Inside was a square white plastic bottle with a white label and black typed letters:

NATALIE GOLDBERG. This was my drug, my medicine. *140 mg. Take three capsules orally once a day. Prescriber: D. Aragon.*

I kept reading. *Caution: Federal law prohibits the transfer of this drug to any person other than the person for whom it was prescribed.* I liked the *for whom.* Someone knew their grammar. But who else would want this? It meant you had cancer. I couldn't give the pills away if I wanted to. And, oh, how badly I wanted to give away the whole catastrophe.

You'd think I'd tear the silver seal off under the cap and pop three in my mouth. I didn't. Instead I peered in. White, big capsules with *ibr* in lowercase printed on each one.

I felt as though I were handling dynamite. Would they work?

I replaced the cap and put the bottle in a kitchen drawer alongside a measuring tape, two candles, a bunch of cards held in a rubber band, three keys, a pile of paper receipts, paper clips, and three unsharpened pencils.

And then I shut the drawer.

Two hours later Yu-kwan came over. "Let me see them." I pointed across the room. "Come with me." She took my hand. I opened the drawer and we peered in together. "Why don't you take the three now?"

I shook my head no. I just couldn't. At least, not yet.

15.

WENDY ARRIVED from California for the second time during my illness. The next day, November 12, she accompanied me to Dulcinea's office in Albuquerque.

I brought a gift for Dulcinea's two-year-old—orange paper butterflies that a student in Ann Arbor had sent me. They were so beautiful that I was never able to bring myself to open them before. Across the chasm of new patient and her doctor, from aging New York Jew to Catholic Albuquerque homegirl thirty years younger, I was trying to make a connection.

I imagined Dulcinea's life: sunk in studies for years, living close to her parents and then, after marriage, also close to her husband's family. She'd shown me photos of her daughter. I leaned over the pictures and admired the small girl wearing glasses, standing tall, her two feet almost together.

I envisioned the pull and delight of being with a young daughter versus the dedication and difficulty of her hard-won profession. The impossibility and hope of saving lives, the victories and defeats. The raw meeting of a patient's fear and need in those small rooms—and, often, the inability to help.

I told Dulcinea all of my reservations about taking ibrutinib. The worst was that, if it didn't work, we wouldn't know for at least three months—and during that time the cancer would keep growing undercover. We discussed the possible side effects: nausea, constipation, diarrhea, muscle aches, and more. In addition, rather than being administered directly into my blood, ibrutinib would run through my digestive system. Mine wasn't so great to begin with. Would it burn out my liver, stomach, intestines?

She heard me out and in the end encouraged me to try the drug anyway. She told me about a patient of hers—a large man, bulked out with tumors. After three months of this drug the results were miraculous, the tumors all gone. "No guarantees, but let's give it a try. Do you have the capsules with you?"

"Yes. In the car." I promised to take them as soon as we left.

With something you want badly, right before you are about to experience it, there is hesitation, resistance.

That's what I felt. The vast unknown offered itself to me—and I was afraid.

Wendy and I dropped in the elevator like a dash in a forgotten sentence, down from the third floor to the ground level. Out the automatic sliding doors into the immense parking lot. It was six minutes till noon. I needed to take the capsules the same time each day. Noon seemed possible. If there was a reaction, it wouldn't keep me up all night, and I wouldn't have to face it first thing in the morning.

Get those things in me and get them working.

But I had to have some ceremony. We walked to my car. At the parking divide was a patch of grass and a spindly tree with no leaves. This spot would have to do.

I knelt down, the three white capsules in my left palm and a water bottle nearby.

First, I spoke to the CLL: "You and I have lived together for a long time."

Wendy whispered, "Twenty-five years."

"It's been long enough. You have to go." The cancer had begun so far back, a silent companion when my beloved teacher died and snaking through the years since. Always with me. Who else can I say that about?

I shook my head and said aloud, "Nat, no more sentiment. Do what you need to."

And then I addressed the ibrutinib, holding up my hand: "Please help me. Do the work you were created for."

I popped those three shiny capsules in my mouth, gulped down water, pressed my lips together, and nodded at Wendy. "Let's go." We got back on I-25 and drove the sixty miles north.

As we drove I looked out the window and asked myself, *Will I cross this street again, see the slant of shadow on this adobe wall, feel the nebulous quality of November— not the beauty of October or the heavy anticipation of December—but November—one more time?* Right then November was the scale for me between life and death.

I hoped the weight would shift, the balance in my favor once again.

CLOSER TO DEATH

On November 19, five days after I ingest my first ibrutinib, I find out that Rima Miller, a woman I knew slightly and who had CLL like me, recently died of complications from the disease. She too had been taking Oh Fat, but after only two infusions she had to quit and needed blood transfusions. On her fifty-ninth birthday she was admitted into Christus St. Vincent Regional Cancer Center's intensive care unit. She never came out alive.

Every person's cancer is different, even if you call it by the same name. Yet Rima's death felt close. A blanket of grief fell over me, my home, the whole street I lived on.

I didn't feel well enough to go to Rima's funeral. But I was told that the synagogue was filled with hundreds of people.

Yu-kwan and I do go to a small ceremony a week later, out at Rima's house, south of town on a mesa with wide-open vistas. She had requested that her body be left on top of Mount Baldy, a high mountain that can be seen from town, especially when covered by snow. She wanted to be feed for wild animals, but that wasn't legal. Instead she was buried in her backyard in a coffin made of reeds, like a big basket. Her grave was dug six feet deep in hard earth during many hours and through the night by her boyfriend. Now it is a big mound covered with crystals, kachinas, colored scarves, an apple, a theater mask, glass beads, and poems friends have left. Over the belly of the grave is a large Middle Eastern rug. At intervals people, unplanned, leave the house and follow the path to where she is lying.

Yu-kwan and I walk out to her grave in late afternoon, clouds low, almost touching the distant mountains. A wind picks up and cuts a cold slash through my winter clothes. The footpath is lined with dozens of standing red roses, a high contrast to the dry terrain. Only on inspection do we realize the roses are artificial. Her boyfriend, who works with props on film crews, planted them. He is kneeling near the head of the grave. I have never met him before. "Thank you for all your effort," I tell him.

He nods and says, *"It's done; we go on."*

I look at Yu-kwan, who is clutching her coat at the collar, grimacing in the cold. She is wearing a thick, dark-blue stocking cap that I know is not warm enough. With the loss of her hair, nothing is warm enough.

Rima's mother and two sisters are buoyed up by all the love and support of people who are connected to Rima. We don't stay long.

The car tires jiggle over the washboard in the uneven dirt road. In that moment. as we drive home, New Mexico feels lonely, basic, vast, grounded only in the excruciating truth of our ultimate end.

16.

TODAY YU-KWAN finally read to me from her journal and showed me her mastectomy scar.

First she read from a small bound notebook:

Ten days ago, my left breast was removed because it had a 3 cm. carcinoma. It looked so perfectly fine on the outside, very much like the right breast that had no abnormalities. My scar looks scary, bumpy, pink, pulled against the flesh as it tries to recover, make whole. I'll never be whole again, losing confidence, feel like everyone is looking at me. The rational Yu-kwan says: It's not like losing a leg or an arm. And, it's still my breast. I am lopsided, a one-winged bird, losing the ability to fly. I always thought that I could handle the worst atrocities, like running away from home, mourning a husband who killed himself, and losing an important relationship. But this is different. I'm helpless after surgery, depending on the kindness of doctors and nurses.

It was a difficult maneuver getting out of bed and the five steps to the toilet. I had to be unplugged from the heart and oxygen monitor, the leg braces to stop blood clots, and the drips. I had to go often and I needed help. Jenna Sue, my night nurse (I called her Nurse Ratchet), did not like me ringing the "N" button. I was in a special ward (not intensive care) but was to be watched every hour. I hardly saw her except at my calling. After a period of waiting, Nurse Sue came grudgingly, impatiently, and in a bad temper. I found myself apologizing, and I was afraid to sleep for fear of what she might do to me or give me. Were the drugs making me paranoid?

I wanted to discharge myself when I thought I had to stay another night because of irregular heartbeats. Fighting or pleading my case for discharge with the doctors and nurses warded off the reality of the missing breast. I've always been healthy. I don't go to the doctors. I didn't have a mammogram for eight years. Yet the last mammogram was clear and it was a self-examination that detected the mass. They called it a palpable mass.

She finally removed the bandages and looked at herself in the mirror—that long horizontal line reaching all the way under her arm. She thought, *Where did my breast go? I don't feel complete anymore.*

"It wasn't so much the physical pain—the pain is emotional. Every time I look at the scar, it's a reminder: I had cancer. Will it come back? With any ache or pain I fear, will it come back?"

Now she unbuttoned her shirt. I'd glanced at her briefly in the bath and shower, but here is her formal presentation. I held my breath. Would I grimace? Could I be supportive?

It looked bad, like a sword had slashed her. I'd seen the famous Deena Metzger poster years ago, of her brazen fantastic display of a tattoo over her mastectomy. This didn't look like that. I immediately hated her surgeon. What was with the extra flap of skin under her left arm?

"Oh, I can see it's still healing." I suggested vitamin E oil. I reached out and touched the scar. Then I touched her single breast.

17.

IT WAS EARLY December, three weeks into my ingestion of ibrutinib. I had the bright idea for us to escape—not that there's any escape—to Florida for a week, right after Yu-kwan's final chemotherapy. We realized it was possible to go, nothing to hold us back. We took the leap.

I was in an old bathing suit, one with splashes of blue flowers. Yu-kwan was tired, not comfortable yet in a bathing suit after her surgery. She sat each day in a front garden near a green lawn, reading the biography of Sonia Sotomayor.

I fluttered by from the pool to the ocean, licking an ice-cream cone. I bent down to kiss her. "Kiss me again," she said, licking her lips, hoping for a taste of ice cream. Her cancer was estrogen positive, thriving on that female hormone, so the doctor told her to avoid dairy. Also sugar and simple carbohydrates. Cancer feeds on them. I was given the same diet. I was eating an ice-cream cone anyway.

Deep down I was sad she could not eat to her heart's delight. No one I'd ever seen—including my fat father, gorging on my grandmother's blintzes, and my friend Eddie, who even ate the reheated food in gas stations, both big men—could outeat Yu-kwan once she got going. I was still astounded that such a petite body could consume so much.

Though she loved the biography she was reading, it was open on her lap, face down, as she relaxed in the shade, watching families saunter by. A young boy with blond curls. A girl dragging a racquet. A grandpa holding an infant wrapped in a light blanket. Occasionally she shaded her eyes with the back of her hand and looked up at the soft southern clouds. She sighed. "America is a beautiful place. Anyplace else"—she was thinking of her childhood—"I could have died of this cancer."

I went to the lap pool, the Atlantic's waves crashing nearby, with that flat even horizon in the distance that goes on forever. Barefoot, looking down at the water, I felt a shift in my body—a sudden space inside, and a tincture of plain happiness spreading through me. *Can this be possible? The ibrutinib is working?* After twenty-one days, maybe it had gained enough accumulated muscle. That powder in each capsule, years of research and thought, experiment, had now reached fruition. The ibrutinib was winning.

I didn't say anything to Yu-kwan.

My energy built through the rest of the week. The morning we were in the Miami airport, about to fly home, I skipped the escalator and bounded up the stairs, my heavy suitcase a mere trinket that I checked in and flung onto the conveyor belt.

When she caught up, Yu-kwan said, "Natalie, it's like you've lost your senses, become manic. Are you okay?"

I only turned up the two corners of my lips and revealed nothing. *Is it really happening?* I didn't want to jinx anything that might be transpiring. I held it all close.

But I was exuberant. The cells in my body were coming alive again, because of that new drug that had been out only a year. While I taught writing students new angles to express what they wanted to say about their mother, sex, toast, their first taste of avocado, researchers in the east of our country were for years relentlessly creating new paths to cut the production of cancer cells in the human body. Thank you, thank you, thank you. You, who I have never acknowledged before.

18.

WHEN I RETURNED home, the exuberance I had felt in Florida dropped completely, as if it had never existed, like a shattered dream. Maybe I was hallucinating in the southern sun?

I saw the oncologist every six weeks, each time getting the dreaded blood test. My blood looked okay, but so what? Last fall it was fine and I had cancer galore.

I was scheduled for another PET scan in February, to see if the drug was working. That big test in the middle of the second full month of winter would tell me the truth. Every ounce of me lived in dread and hope.

I fantasized endlessly what I would do if I was clear. How I would get in my old car, the one I loved—the navy Volvo station wagon with the wide seats and turbo engine. I would travel the empty boundless Midwest, stopping in small, lost, sometimes suspicious towns. These would be dark American places where my Jewish genes were not allowed but places that mirrored my own boundless emptiness. I also imagined showing Yu-kwan Big Sur, driving down along the high cliffs at the edge of the Pacific, the big water stretching to Japan, where I also planned to go and follow the trail of Basho, the great seventeenth-century haiku writer. Oh, I had plans. Over to Paris, gaze again at Monet's water lilies, drink hot chocolate at Les Deux Magots. Come back to the States and follow the rough coast of Maine, go again to Grandma and Grandpa's graves in Elmont, New York. Drive to the tip of Long Island and swim in the brown Atlantic. Go to Canio's, the poetry bookstore in Sag Harbor, where they sell poetry books by Mr. Clemente, my ninth-grade English teacher.

I wanted to see the Art Institute of Chicago, eat at Detroit's Greek restaurants, for the first time behold Birmingham's Civil Rights National Memorial. Go to the Phillips Collection in DC, then over to Fort Worth's water park, the hamburger shop on the corner with the red-checked tablecloths, visit again the city's three art museums, right in a row, on the same street. The Amon Carter, the Kimball, the Modern. I'd walk from one museum to another, getting a strong whiff of the stockyards a mile off. Then the Oregon coast, Seattle, Vancouver, Mill Valley's library, and the lettuce fields at Green Gulch. I wanted to spread my happy no-cancer arms over the whole universe.

I would abruptly stop those rolling thoughts. I didn't know what the results would be. I didn't know anything. That was the truth.

And beyond anticipation, in a much more primal place, fear raged. It bowled through me, uncontrolled. No meditation, yoga stance, massage, deep breathing, allayed its force. All I could do was acknowledge it, realize it was innate. On an animal level, we all want to survive.

February 17 was D-day for getting the PET scan. While I waited for that day to come, in my restless, nervous impatience, I painted two self-portraits. Each time I'd look over the sink into the mirror and say, talking to the pen in my hand, "Make me pretty." Then I'd make the initial sketch. I'd draw quickly, place the pad on the table and look down at the sheet of paper. Was that me—at the edge of fury, hysteria, madness? That's not what I saw in the mirror, but on the page a more unvarnished reality stared back.

I grabbed for the brush and dipped it in a light cadmium green, the color of split pea soup, and painted the whites of my eyes, changed them to the color of terror. I painted purple on the haunted, bruised cheekbones, a pale pink mouth, slightly opened in stunned recognition, hair streaked in orange, bare branches in the background.

A week later I tried another self-portrait. *Pretty* was not in my hand's vocabulary. I had to accept the raw emotions on my face. In life it was harder. I was living them.

I took the three ibrutinib pills each day at noon. I also did normal things: got my hair cut, went to acupuncture appointments, met Miriam and Susana for lunch, had my teeth cleaned, visited with my friend Sean Murphy from Taos, even went to a talk on James Baldwin at the Lensic Theater downtown. But whatever I did, I lived for one thing: the results of taking those pills for three months. If they weren't working, the cancer would be further along—and I would be closer to death.

The day finally came. Susana drove me down to Albuquerque in her yellow car. I hadn't slept at all the night before. My muscles ached, and a headache was forming over my left eye. The miles of sagebrush we passed through looked dry and desolate. No snow. Bare ground.

As usual, the lab tech in the Cancer Center couldn't find a vein. She was inexperienced, and after two tries I asked for someone else. Her replacement, a young man who didn't smile, managed to shoot the nuclear sugar into my veins. The big crazy machine snapped pictures while my body slid back and forth inside like a ham on a conveyor belt.

Afterward, I fell back into the waiting room. I found Susana, and we drove straight home.

As soon as I got inside the front door I stripped off my clothes, dropped them on the floor, and got under the bedsheets. It was just after noon. I lay there staring up at the ceiling for much of the rest of the day.

Originally I was scheduled to see Dulcinea the next day to go over the results. But the week before, the center had called and rescheduled our appointment for Friday, three days after the test. I tried to explain to the woman how much stress was involved in a longer wait, but she was curt: "I'm sorry." And hung up.

I was indignant, called her back. That changed nothing. Once again I had to accept that I was not in control. I was contending with the big industrial machine of American health care. (I learned later that Dulcinea knew nothing about this switch.)

So, instead, the day after the PET scan, I took comfort in not knowing the results. I had all day Wednesday and Thursday to bask in ignorance. A part of me understood the verdict was already in—whatever was happening in my body had been happening in my body for a while. But on Friday my conscious mind would meet my body's performance. It had been responding—or not responding—to ibrutinib for months.

So on that knowledge-free Wednesday afternoon I was painting a car green—I'd stopped the self-portraits—and the car was slowly morphing to blue. I planned to call it *Homage to California* because I drew the car at my friend Helen's home in Palo Alto. It was an old Rambler

Ambassador with flat tires that I saw in someone's driveway every time I visited her. I'd attempted to draw it before, but the sketches never worked. I'd almost given up. But one morning I woke early, marched out there in my pajamas with great determination, and did a new sketch. Even though it wasn't a perfect rendition, I caught its spirit. Now, many months later, I was finally painting it.

The phone rang. It was Erica, my primary care doctor. She had a spring in her voice. "Natalie!"

I gripped the paintbrush tightly. I knew she had my results. I'd given the nuclear department her fax number but had forgotten. My heart was banging in my chest.

"It's good. It's good," she said.

"Tell me! Tell me!"

"See if you can take this in." She read from the report, "'The bones have dramatic decrease of the multifocal metabolic activity.'"

"Is that good? Is that good?"

"Wait. Listen. 'The previously described hypermetabolic lymph node activity has resolved.'"

I was trembling. I heard fragments: "'no longer avid . . . no longer pathologically enlarged.'"

"Erica, tell me—what?"

"Nat, it's very, very good. That drug is a miracle. The cancer is gone."

"Really? Really?"

"You'll see your oncologist and go over everything. She'll explain. Nat, congratulations."

"Yippee!" I yelled, like a cowgirl. We hung up.

Outside the window above my painting table, the aspens cast long shadows across the fence. I stood up, hugged myself, and grabbed for the phone.

First I called Yu-kwan. "I do not have cancer. Nothing lit up. I can't talk. Come over."

Then I called almost everyone I knew. In each call I repeated those first two essential lines, then said, "I have to go," hung up, and dialed the next person. After that I paced my studio, then the house for several minutes. Finally I careened into the backyard in a thin T-shirt, talking to myself among the frozen fruit trees.

I finished the Rambler painting a few days later. The car was big, fat, and ready to roll. I changed its title to *Happiness*.

• • •

On Friday, knowing the results, I drove down with Annie to see Dulcinea, who had a bad cold, caught from her young daughter.

"Her dad, her grandma and grandpa, all have it," she explained. "We couldn't stay away from holding, cuddling, kissing her." She was wearing a white mask to protect her patients, so her usual expressive face was hidden, but her eyebrows popped up and down as she talked. I could feel her deep satisfaction at the results.

She reminded me that, though the results were good and there was no sign of cancer now, I had a chronic condition, "Someday," she said, "the cancer will figure a way around the ibrutinib." I had to continue to take the pills as maintenance, but no one knew how long the drug would continue to work. A year, two, three? It was still a new drug, and each person's cancer is different.

She told me that the radiologist, who analyzed hundreds of scans, remembered the test from four months ago, and she couldn't believe the new results. My insides, which had been drenched in cancer, were no longer pathologically enlarged.

I couldn't believe it either. It was as though I'd been kidnapped, with death like a sharp knife swinging constantly over my head, and then suddenly flown back home. I identified with Iraqi war veterans—the change was so sudden.

I was supposedly normal again, as if no hole had been blown through the center of my life.

19.

DURING THE WEEKS that followed, I thought a lot about my parents, reaching back to when I was young. How my father carried loneliness, the same way another person carried his royalty or her athleticism. His loneliness was big, broad, and open. He sat in the middle of it, never trying to break its spell, never struggling outside its circumference. It didn't have a grip on him, exactly because he didn't fight it, didn't deny its place in the human plentitude. Even in the middle of family gatherings, with all of his blood relatives from Brooklyn at our dinner table, he was in an independent sea.

My father faced one of life's truths squarely, and because of that there was an authority about him, a wisdom—and a plague. People were afraid of him, of what he'd say because he was fearless. His second shoe had already dropped; he was no longer trying to defend something, keep up appearances, be someone.

I'm not sure how he came to this, but seeing it all of my life had a potent influence. I wanted that freedom. Maybe fighting in the war, or the rejection of his orthodox Jewish parents, or the opening of the camps—that a human life could be considered worthless—effected his brooding single distrust, his wariness. But it also created a humanizing independence. I remembered him when I was a child—he'd become a champion swimmer in high school—using the crawl to go farther out than anyone was allowed to at Jones Beach, into the rough salty expanse.

My mother was just the opposite. She could not face her sorrow, never attempted to turn around and see what was chasing her. In and out of the discount stores, every single day, searching for peace in a blouse, for happiness in the right dress or shoe or tablecloth. Who could blame her? There was no guide into a promised land. The woman ached—a terrible disappointment engulfed her, and I beheld it. The harder it pushed, the faster she ran into the brand-new, hopeful discount megastore they built on Long Island. No driving distance was too great. Her foot on the gas pedal and the windows opened in the humid summers.

What was her sadness? I could give a litany. She was smart, but no one thought of sending her to college. She loved color, pattern, texture, but her only outlet was in the endless rows of store clothes. The man she really loved, Eddie Smith, the next-door neighbor, forsook her after he came home from the war. My father was found on the rebound, sitting in a hammock on his brother Sam's rundown estate in Bay Shore. My mother's parents were renting a summer cottage on the premises. What is love anyway? You recognize the loneliness in someone else or the hope of losing it with them.

I saw the outlandish connection of my mother and father, one of those couples that never belonged together. She wanted riches; he was happy with two pairs of shorts. She only cared about what others thought; he never gave thought to another's needs. But now I saw something I never understood before. In the song of the world, they contained each other, kept each other in check. They weren't happy, but in the hollow of my father, my mother's unattainable peace was held in place, like a lock clicked shut. One twisted to the left; one to the right. In this way they balanced each other.

On a Tuesday at 3:00 a.m., deep under the covers but unable to sleep, listening to the tap of bare branches against the windowpane, the endless tick of the clock on the nightstand, trying to trace and make sense of my life, I saw that I carried their suffering in my own cells, compounded by my own. Where were my parents now? Gone. Where will I be? Gone.

How to make the best of my time left?

Who am I? *Quickly, quickly, without thinking, what is*

159

your original face before your parents were born? Whole continents have never heard of a Zen koan, this puzzle revealing truth. Still, the dilemma continues. How to live when the ground has been taken away. No more mother or father, no more energy of youth, no more dream of infallibility. No more health.

The wind is blowing hard outside. The sun high and full. Three times I have applied lip balm in the last two hours. Dry with no promise of rain.

Earlier today I went to a class on William Faulkner's *Light in August*. Whatever he wrote, whatever agony he lived, whatever prize he won, he too is gone. Sure we remember him, but where is William Faulkner?

ENDLESSLY LIKE A RIVER

When visiting Rome, any former English major in their right mind must go to the non-Catholic cemetery for foreigners, Via Caio Cestio. John Keats, the Romantic poet who died at age twenty-six, rumored to be a virgin, is buried here. So is Percy Shelley.

Forty-two years after graduating from college, as I walk down the rows of stones looking for Keats, "Ode on a Grecian Urn" blooms in me all over again. *Heard melodies are sweet, but those unheard / are sweeter . . . Thou, silent form! dost tease us out of thought / as doth eternity.*

As I place a stone and say thank you, my young, sincere love of literature returns. I meet not only Keats but young Natalie again.

I walk farther. I'd heard rumors that the poet Gregory Corso ended up here too. I met him when I studied with Allen Ginsberg in the seventies. I'd read in a newspaper that in his last months he was cared for by his daughter in Saint Paul, Minnesota, that straight-laced Midwestern city on the Mississippi. So unlike crazy Gregory.

Down the line of stones and Italian cypresses, I find the poet Shelley's grave. And then, stuck at an odd angle right up front, I see a stone for Corso. His daughter managed to bring his ashes and bury them here.

At seventeen Gregory was the youngest prisoner ever to be in maximum security in Clinton, New York, on three counts: stealing a suit to go to a wedding, sleeping in his teacher's room, and, the final straw, stealing a toaster. The previous inhabitant in the cell was the Mafioso Lucky Luciano, who also showed the Allies a way into Italy through Sicily. Luciano had left all of his books behind.

In that cell, Corso discovered Shelley. As he turned in the direction of poetry, his life was saved, and he always wished to be buried near his great master, that Romantic poet.

On Corso's stone, I read:

> Spirit
> is Life
> it flows thru
> the death of me
> endlessly
> like a river
> unafraid
> of becoming
> the sea

What else to say? All in that Corso poem.

20.

MARCH 1, A SUNDAY, was Katagiri Roshi's twenty-fifth memorial day. Yu-kwan and I went to a concert at three in the afternoon to hear Midori, the famous Japanese violinist. Our seats were up close. She was a small woman who had a big sound. I watched her bend and sway in a loose-fitting, short-sleeved black-and-white dress. The music seemed to come up through her hips and legs; it was as if the violin played her. A thin string from the bow suddenly snapped and dangled. She didn't stop. She and the violin played on into the ocean of Schumann.

I thought of my teacher, twenty-five years dead. That's a long time. How could I have been so lucky? His lectures every Saturday morning and Wednesday night—I never understood most of what he said, but my body drank it, took it all in. And when he died at sixty-two and we sat for three days with his corpse in the zendo, my body also took this in. I could not accept his death.

Four months ago, right before I went under the anesthesia for the stent surgery, I whispered *thank you*, and I saw my young body sitting still by the window in the zendo. All of his effort to bring Zen to the United States—out of the war, and Hiroshima, Nagasaki, General MacArthur—to that white room by a lake in Minnesota. What was I doing there?

Even in art history class in college, when the professor showed slides of exceptional architecture in Minnesota—the IDS building by Mies van der Rohe, the bank in Owatonna by Louis Sullivan—I took exceptional note. I had no idea at that time who I was or where I was going, but I knew that Minneapolis was in my destiny.

I'd never used the word *destiny* before. What is it? A coagulation of your hunger to find a path, to find a place, to set one foot after another. To come inside out; to show your guts, everything you are made of.

If this was true about destiny, cancer was my ally on that course. It pushed me out beyond any boundary I had known. It threw me right into the pool of fear, stripped me down to animal survival. Could I face that polarity of life and death and find another place to stand?

· · ·

Tears rolled down Yu-kwan's face. Schumann was one of her favorite composers.

Her hair was growing in slowly and looked like duckling fuzz, very, very short. She felt self-conscious, didn't realize she was now fashionable, hip, wearing big earrings.

After the concert, as we walked across Santa Fe Plaza, a tall, handsome man in his twenties ran after her, then walked backward to face her after he caught up. "Excuse me," he said, shy but determined. "I just want to tell you—I love your hair."

Yu-kwan lit up. "Thank you." I could tell she felt beautiful again.

What has cancer taught me? How old will I be when I die? I didn't know. I settled on seventy-five. Then I decided on eighty-six.

Over the summer, when I was receiving infusions, I'd heard on the radio that Peter Matthiessen, Zen teacher and author of *The Snow Leopard*, plus many other books, died on a Saturday at eighty-six. On the following Monday his last novel came out. The novel was the conclusion of his struggle to comprehend, make peace with Auschwitz. Years earlier, I sat opposite him along the railroad tracks at that concentration camp during a weeklong retreat. Now I thought, *Yes, that's how a writer should die, writing to the last.* Eighty-six gave me a hopeful number.

No one knows when their death will come; I remember the words Katagiri said that one December in the zendo.

21.

YU-KWAN AND I were both now on the other side of cancer—at least for now. A possible return loomed over us. And we found ourselves alienated from each other.

Taking care of our individual cancers worked well, but now we didn't know how to come together again. She had become a stranger.

We went through the motions of dinner together, a movie, maybe a walk. We didn't say much—we never talked a lot together, but before, our silence was weighty, full of feeling, contentment, and trust. Now it felt like a wafer we kept cracking and crumbling with each step.

And I knew a good heart-to-heart would not work. It was never our way. I felt lonesome and sad, but I had no energy or inspiration to adjust our connection. I thought, *We are falling apart, breaking up right before our eyes, and neither one of us can do anything about it.* We went through the motions of a relationship, our roots underground grappling to reach each other.

One Saturday morning, in an effort to break through, she showed up with a gift, a small box she presented to me. I opened it. Fancy clip-on (I've never pierced my ears) turquoise earrings from an upscale tourist shop on the Plaza.

I'd lived in New Mexico for forty years. I already had all the turquoise I'd ever need. I didn't want these.

I tried them on. They looked awful. I thought, *She has no understanding of me.*

I took them off, handed them back. Through gritted teeth I said, "Can you return them?"

Her eyes were cast down. "Yes, I asked before I bought them. We can have credit."

"Well, thanks anyway." I was as cold as an outdoor winter doorknob.

She looked at me. If eyes could cut, I would be sliced to pieces.

· · ·

Two days later, when I woke up, I felt a splash of happiness. For no reason I thought, *I'll roast a chicken.* What a good idea. Potatoes, carrots, a salad. I didn't think: *Oh, now things will be good.* I just took one step after another— bought the poultry, rubbed paprika, garlic, salt, pepper into the skin the way my grandmother taught me. The roasting aroma filled the kitchen, and I hummed as I tore lettuce leaves.

I invited Yu-kwan. An hour later I heard the click of the front door. She entered the kitchen. "Smells great." She went to the shelf, reached for two plates, pulled out forks and knives, set the table in an old rhythm we had established before the cancer.

The meal was ready. We sat down and dug in.

"This meat is so juicy," Yu-kwan said as we ate. "I like the dressing this time."

After dinner we relaxed. We had shifted to another dimension—one we couldn't find before through struggle or discussion. Our bodies had to shift out of fear, out of the physical onslaught we'd been through. This couldn't be pushed, manipulated.

Cancer taught me I wasn't in control.

Really though, I'd learned that before—from falling in love. A turn of dark hair, noticing someone's shyness, can flip you into that realm.

To truly find our way back to each other, we had to let go, follow a circuitous route. Our will had little to do with it.

22.

IN LATE SPRING, Yu-kwan and I took the hiking trip in Ireland that we had canceled the year before. Both of us were up and able but also a bit baffled, like two people let out of a dark prison into the light. Would we hold up? It wasn't a group tour. We would be going it alone, with maps and accommodations set up ahead of time by a company in Vancouver. Just the two of us. No connections, no one we knew in Ireland. And after Ireland we planned to fly to Yorkshire and hike the Dales. In all, we would be gone almost a month.

As we headed out on rocky paths, up and down hills, as trial runs, my hip hurt, then my left shoulder. Each time I was sure the cancer had returned. Pain amplified the fear.

On the third morning, I panicked. "We made a terrible mistake. We need to fly home immediately." But we didn't. Instead, we waited for the taxi that the Vancouver company had arranged to pick us up and take us to the trailhead, for a seven-mile hike ending by the sea. It had rained hard the night before, and it was still drizzling.

The beginning of the hike was a cold, dismal spot. Through the fog we saw a marker up ahead. I was wearing a pink slicker; Yu-kwan, behind me, was wearing a gray poncho. Underneath we were bundled up with woolen clothes.

We came to a bramble crowding against a huge puddle. I managed to edge along it and get to the other side. As I did, I heard a big splash. I turned to see Yu-kwan flat supine in the middle of the puddle.

I gasped. "Are you okay? What happened? Do you want to go back?"

She lifted herself up. "No. Let's keep going." She shook herself off.

I smiled as I forged ahead. *I love that girl*, I thought, and from then on the balance was tipped. No matter what fear or hesitation arose, I kept saying, *Let it go, Nat.* And I did.

The next day we took an old fishing boat to the Aran Islands and walked five miles against a strong wind to our guesthouse. For breakfast each morning I ate Irish porridge, and it sustained me, seemed to settle my overexcited stomach. We took pictures. We chatted with locals. I read a novel called *Grief* by Andrew Holleran that I had brought from the States. It dipped me back into sadness, reminded me that no matter how cheerful Yu-kwan and I became, the blast of the last fourteen months was continually at our backs.

On the last morning, we were dropped off in the Connemara, an area of big mountains with little vegetation. Even the cab driver gasped when he saw where he had taken us. We had to climb a steep mountain to get to a path on the other side. No houses, nothing anywhere. Only some scraggly sheep and goats.

I got out of the back seat slowly. "Are you sure this is right?"

He nodded. "This is what the directions say."

We took a few breaths. The cab turned around and drove off along the stony road.

Yu-kwan and I looked at each other, then up at the incline. I raised my shoulders in resignation. "Might as well." I've never climbed anything as steep. Near the top was supposed to be a small chapel to Saint Francis. The rumor was that he passed through here once.

We finally reached what looked like the top, only to discover it was merely a hump. The incline continued. My calves ached. There was no going back, nothing to go back to—only a rocky, empty landscape spread behind us. In front of us were piles of sharp slate. We had to balance and step from one pile to another.

Sweat running down our faces, we finally reached the top. The promised chapel was there, and we collapsed near the small altar outside.

I opened my pack and we munched a few nuts and raisins, too tired to eat the bread we had brought from breakfast.

"I'm praying." Yu-kwan dragged herself over to the altar. Who cares what religion? We were ready to prostrate ourselves in humility. We had made it this far.

When she was done, I stumbled over and knelt down. *Please let my life continue. Let me live. Saint Francis, you of the birds and nature and poverty, please give me life.*

It was a sharp steep downhill climb, more difficult than up. My legs shook.

A baby lamb ran across the path. I watched it as I walked—and fell hard on my knees and hands. The slate cut through my pants.

"Are you okay?" Yu-kwan shrieked.

"I think so." There was a gash on my knee and my left palm was scraped hard. No bandages, no phone, no people, no help.

We staggered down the rest of the hill to a high iron fence with no way around. We'd have to climb it. I threw my pack over.

On the first try I couldn't lift my bruised knee high enough. The thought ran through me: *This is what you get for praying to a Christian saint.* I tried again—standing near the top rung, I lifted my other knee first. It worked. I hoisted myself over to the other side.

A long uninhabited dirt road was ahead. The map said ten more miles.

After three miles we heard a car in the distance. I thought, *No, my knee can make it.* But as the small white car neared, I shot out my hand and waved. The car stopped beside us.

"Climb in. Where you going?

"Amazing I'm here. I would never come this way, but me sister needs me to pick up her children from school. She just called." The driver repeated this twice as we bumped along.

We told him where we came from, that we just climbed over that mountain where the chapel was.

"Is it still in good shape? Twenty-five years ago, me and another man built it. Took us a long time. We had to carry up all the equipment."

I'm sitting in the back, my leg propped up along the length of the seat; I lean forward. "You built it? You were the person?"

"Me and another fellow." He shook his head. "Of course, we were younger then."

I lay back against the window. The old saint did hear my prayers. *Thank you*, I whispered.

23.

AFTER IRELAND we flew to Yorkshire, England, where Yu-kwan once lived. We stayed in a guesthouse for a week near the famous Yorkshire Dales—hundreds of miles of trails, starting from the Lake District up north and through national parks. We went out each day to hike to small country towns along the River Wharfe.

In England, depression took root in me, spread through my limbs, blackened my blood, and dragged me down. I was mystified by it. How come? Wasn't I in the swing of things now, having a great time?

The English air pierced through my woolen jacket, even in May. We passed through turnstiles, fences, gates, and farms. The river to my left ran over rocks and wound through the countryside, like in a Corot painting. Small trees, hazy with new leaves, were shadowed by dead, dark-black oaks. It was law, even written in the Magna Carta, that people should be able to walk through private property, passing through gates and fields. Occasionally we passed a couple, or a group of jolly older people, fit and healthy.

It was lambing season. All along the trail in the pastures, scruffy sheep were birthing lambs, small enough to tuck in a daypack. As we passed by three large stones, following a curve—behold! A tiny black lamb, just popped out, stood on our path, stunned, motionless. That soft vulnerability, that tentative melting transparent presence stopped me dead, sliced through my heavy heart. My depression crumbled in the presence of such radiance.

The next morning, depression flooded me again. But this time I didn't bludgeon myself and wrestle with it, grab and manufacture every painful memory I could. I let it all be—and, like a mist, by late morning it dissolved.

The next morning the same thing. I'd known this from Zen. Don't solidify. Don't feed your thoughts. Allow all and everything to pass through. I had to discover it all over again.

The last day, we took a leap and rented a car—the steering wheel on the right, us driving on the left, English style. On narrow country roads, everything shifted to opposites. As we barreled out of the hotel that early morning, my instincts kicked in. I was careening merrily down the right—but now wrong—side of the road, staring at the green fields and stone walls. All at once a big silver Mercedes came at us. I honked the horn, indignant. *Get on the left.* Then, in a flash, *Get over, Nat.* The Mercedes slowed enough that I saw the gaping mouths of the couple inside, their disbelief at my arrogance. They probably surmised: *Americans.*

We were off to Haworth, an hour away, to visit the parsonage and home of the Brontë sisters. Three members of the family had died early, their mother from cancer and two sisters from typhus. Their minister father buried the three in the family vault at the parsonage. The remaining daughters consoled themselves with writing, often with their brother, creating wild fantasies, sometimes carried to the verge of insanity. But eventually the three sisters matured and settled around an oak dining room table, each working diligently on a story. After dinner they'd walk around the table, commenting on each other's work. The sisters had little formal education except writing, writing, writing together at that table. These stories in the end became Emily's *Wuthering Heights*, Charlotte's *Jane Eyre*, Anne's *Agnes Grey* and *The Tenant of Wildfell Hall.* World-famous novels. Their creative lives flourished in each other's company, close to the untamed land that was such an inspiration for them.

Yu-kwan and I stood a long time gazing into the dining room at that table. I'd spent my whole life teaching writing practice, encouraging people in small groups to do timed writing. It felt as though these young women sitting at this table after dinner—since they were five years old till their deaths, always writing—invented writing practice. And here was the original table where it all began in the early eighteen hundreds. I was mesmerized.

Afterward, we hiked the moors, miles behind the house, to the waterfalls where the sisters often went.

All the directional signs on the moor were in English and Japanese. The Japanese study the Brontë sisters in school and come to this island country on the other side of the planet to pay homage.

A group of thirty secondary students, visiting from Paris, chaperones in tow, was hiking ahead of us. At the crossing in the creek they stopped for lunch. We caught up and sat on the other side. When they left, we watched two young students linger and make out with all the power of first passion.

After the French students left, we were alone on the literary heath. We took the steeper climb to windswept Top Withens, a ruined farmhouse, which was where Emily placed the Earnshaw family house in *Wuthering Heights*—then, farther on, to the rock where Cathy and Heathcliffe met.

The Brontë sisters' beloved brother, Branwell, died suddenly at thirty-one, a year after his sisters' novels were published under pseudonyms. Soon after, Emily and Anne contracted tuberculosis. Emily never left the parsonage again, dying in December 1848 at age thirty.

Anne, anxious to try a sea cure, set out with Charlotte for Scarborough several months after Emily's death, where she died four days later at the age of twenty-nine. To spare her father the anguish of another family funeral, Charlotte had her sister buried by the sea and then returned to Haworth alone.

Charlotte lived to publish two more novels. She married her father's curate and, less than a year later, died at thirty-eight in the early stages of pregnancy. Outliving his wife and all of his children, Patrick Brontë died at the age of eighty-four.

I asked around. The local Haworth public schools did not read their famous authors, the Brontë sisters. The same in Ireland: I was told students there did not read James Joyce. It was an old story. We don't recognize the greatness in front of us. We all long for another story, another place.

I was sixty-seven years old. That's a lot more years than the Brontës lived. Sixty-seven is a long time. How lucky I was.

24.

THAT NIGHT, I sat in a window seat overlooking a valley. Yu-kwan was lying in bed, reading a book. I asked her, "Did you think you were going to die when you had cancer?"

She drew her head out of the pages. Until this moment, we hadn't dared talk about it, even though it hovered around us all the time. "I wanted to last as long as I could. I worried so. There was a point—you didn't know it—but we almost lost you. When there was a chance the CLL was morphing into something else. I've only prayed three times in my life, and that was one of them."

"Really?" I gulped, tried to take it in. *I almost died?* Sure, I knew it but repressed it as soon as I could.

"Where would you have wanted your ashes?" I asked. "I never even asked—I assume you want a cremation."

Yu-kwan sat up in bed. "For sure. But if I'm dead and only ashes, who cares where they go?"

"I care. I can't decide where I'd want my ashes though. Maybe near Katagiri Roshi's zendo on the bluffs of the Mississippi. Some of his are there. You can have friends take them different places. You can designate it in your will, even leave money for their travel. I thought of some at the Artist's Cemetery in Woodstock, near Milton Avery's grave; some out at the tip of Long Island, where Jackson Pollock is buried. It's an awfully pretty place, and Betty Friedan and Hannah Wilke are there too—"

"Who's Hannah Wilke?" Yu-kwan was alert now. "I want my ashes next to yours."

"She's the feminist who sculpted clay vaginas. Then there's the Jewish cemetery up in Taos—or at Upaya Zen Center, if they start having a burial ground. A little with my family at the Hebrew cemetery in Elmont, near Belmont racetrack."

"You've got a lot of places."

"Maybe Paris, Yosemite—it's hard to choose one. Fuck it, I don't want to die."

"You'll exhaust your friends." We start to laugh.

What we did talk a lot about during the cancer was our wills. Someone slighted us—we took them out; someone left a roast chicken at the door and we put them in. At one point the mailman left three great letters in one day. I was ready to leave all of my assets to the U.S. Postal Service.

Yu-kwan, who loved noodles but couldn't eat them anymore—too many carbs—declared that the noodle place, where she often ate, on the East Side of Manhattan would get her estate. They could feed the homeless.

Then we wondered: Would there be anything left? Neither of us was working. The cancer twins might go out starving.

25.

IT IS AUGUST 13. Kids in Abiquiú, New Mexico, are going back to school today. I feel sad for these kids, already tucked back into desks in rows. They should have a full dose of summer, of verdant shadows, the play of night crickets, bare feet, shorts, striped T-shirts, lake water against skin, hours of boredom, using a stick to draw in the dirt. Is this all a fantasy of a summer long gone? I don't care. Everyone should taste no ambition, no goal, the big sky, and the dark cliffs.

I have often driven out alone this summer from Santa Fe, fifty minutes away, to swim in Abiquiu Lake. I come out here by myself to dive into this water near the Pedernal, the flat-top flint mountain that Georgia O'Keeffe repeatedly painted in the forties—her ashes on top—its wide flanks spreading to the east like a great embrace.

I am supposed to be working on a book, but the Rio Chama is dammed into a blue lake in the desert against pink cliffs, and I can't stay away. Summer is water—and swimming.

I had the privilege—I only understand that now—of spending many Julys and Augusts at the beach on Long Island, where I rode the forever-crashing waves, clinging to my father's bare shoulders. This summer, after my year of cancer, I want more than ever to be by water.

Now I am driving back home, windows rolled down, in the late afternoon in my wet bathing suit. I swing into the Bode's parking lot, the only store in the area. It was here even when Georgia was, back in the forties, when the local young called her Miss O'Keeffe. It's a combination grocery and café, selling fishing equipment, souvenir cards, sunhats, sunscreen. Out front, piled high, is a huge supply of twenty-five-pound bags of sunflower seeds, which people lug home to feed wild birds.

At the back of the parking lot, near large shady cottonwoods, is a tiny shack, painted white with a sign: MR. FROSTY'S MALTS, SHAKES, CONES. And a banner hung from two poles: DREYER'S ICE CREAM. I like that brand. *I shouldn't have it on my cancer diet* crosses my mind for the slightest moment. I step up to the window, the only person there, and order one scoop of butter pecan and one of coffee, in a cup. I pay my $4.50—a fair price if you've eaten at those gourmet gelato places.

I sit down with my white plastic spoon and dig in.

It's just the right chill and consistency, so it won't melt before I'm done—and I won't be done for a while.

I take small mouthfuls; I want this to last. The butter pecan, a lighter beige, shot through with nuts, balances atop the darker beige of the coffee scoop. Proust and his madeleine have nothing on me. His cookie coalesces the past, but this ice cream lands me in the exquisite present. Where else would I want to be?

In this moment, I use the truth of death to my advantage, as leverage, an edge into this delicious present. How many more? Only this one spoonful at a time into my mouth, this best wet summer in forty years in this Land of Enchantment.

The coffee shocks my tongue after the less directed flavor of butter pecan. I am ready for it. No regrets. I down every morsel.

No worry about calories. This is my one heavenly life. This afternoon. This Thursday. This sun on the pale dirt and the cottonwood green leaves. This blue mesa in the distance, this gutsy temporary life lived as the Buddha taught—with gusto.

AFTERWORD

OF ALL THE painters I love, Pierre Bonnard is my secret favorite, the one I catch out of the corner of my eye, acknowledge again and again.

You cannot stamp his work into memory. Instead, his paintings move through you in waves. Color on color on color. I have seen this same sentiment expressed in interviews with other painters. When asked about their influences, they name a few. Then the interviewer mentions Bonnard. Oh yes, yes, of course him.

A few weeks after he finally married Marthe, his long-time muse, Renée Monchaty, his live model and mistress, committed suicide. For years afterward he painted Marthe in the bath, often in a deep tub of water. Though the paintings are beautiful, they also look haunted, like someone reclining in a sarcophagus. His late interiors give an initial impression of domestic contentment, but looked at carefully, they suggest disquiet, a lack of presence, an emotional absence of human fulfillment. Bonnard was silently grieving through the medium of paint.

I do not visit Bonnard's grave. But twice—once in Paris and once at the Legion of Honor museum in San Francisco—I viewed the last piece he painted, a week before his death in 1947. *Almond Tree in Blossom*. Full of light. The tree in white takes over most of the canvas, and it feels as though it were about to ascend. It almost glitters.

When Japanese Zen masters approach death, they write a last poem to reveal their mind at the final moment. In this final painting, Bonnard does something similar, displays his lightening heart. Before the great question—How is it to live with eternity at your door?—Bonnard answers: In full bloom.

MEDITATION ON METTA

THIS IS the Loving-Kindness Chant (version by Maylie Scott) that I recited on the pier in the first chapter.

> May I be well, loving, and peaceful.
> May all beings be well, loving, and peaceful.
> May I be at ease in my body, feeling the ground
> beneath my seat and feet, letting my back be
> long and straight, enjoying breath as it rises
> and falls and rises.
>
> May I know and be intimate with body-mind,
> whatever its feeling or mood, calm or agitated,
> tired or energetic, irritated or friendly.
> Breathing in and out, in and out, aware, moment
> by moment, of the risings and passings.
>
> May I be attentive and gentle toward my own
> discomfort and suffering.

May I be attentive and grateful for my own joy and well-being.

May I move toward others freely and with openness.

May I receive others with sympathy and understanding.

May I move toward the suffering of others with peaceful and attentive confidence.

May I recall the Bodhisattva of Compassion, her one thousand hands, her instant readiness for action. Each hand with an eye in it, the instinctive knowing what to do.

May I continually cultivate the ground of peace for myself and others and persist, mindful and dedicated to this work, independent of results.

May I know that my peace and the world's peace are not separate; that our peace in the world is a result of our work for justice.

May all beings be well, happy, and peaceful.

ACKNOWLEDGMENTS

Thank you, Susan Voorhees, who brought dinner every Tuesday night for more than a year; Upaya Zen Center, whose members fed me and were generally available while I had cancer; Jane Steinberg, who dropped off little boxes of perfectly planned macrobiotic meals; Rob Strell and Gary McAfee, who brought a whole dressed turkey for Thanksgiving, fresh from the oven with all the fixings, in the trunk of their car from Albuquerque; and Rob, who left at my door a perfect basket of spring apricots from his tree. Thank you to Mirabai Starr for her lamb stew; cousin Elizabeth Jacobson for the fat, hot roast chickens she delivered often; Onde Chymes for her special oxtail soup; Mary Feidt for her pie and Eddie Lewis for delivering it and for accompanying me to a biopsy and being a general support; Kitchen Angels for delivering meals; Katie Arnold, who insisted I walk, even if just down the road, and brought me smoothies she made with Maisy, her four-year-old; Mark Little and David Gardner for the brownies and the last-minute delivery of Mexican dinners; Rob Wilder for chicken and home-cooked pinto beans; Miriam Sagan for the organic squash dish; Joan Baker for hiring Bonnie Lynch to make homemade quick-frozen chicken soups; Bonnie Paul—I'll never forget the barbecued ribs; Susan York for her lemon tart. I know some of this sounds like a gourmet feast, but fourteen months is a lot of meals, and food is always important. Thank you, thank you, thank you.

A special thanks to Wendy Johnson, Susana Guillaume, and Annie Lewis for their personal care and support throughout; my sister Romi Goldberg for her support over the phone and the gift she sent; Joan Halifax, who visited me almost every day and always had my back; Genzan Quennell, who hooked up my computer to read test results at UNM; Carol Soutor, who stayed on top of medical research while at the same time tending to her dying sister, Ruth Albrecht Soutor; Dr. Erica Elliott, who e-mailed me encouragement every single morning of my illness; Ann Filemyr for going with me to the first oncologist appointment at UNM; Michele Huff for coming to the oncologist with me on several last-minute occasions; Sean Murphy and Tania Casselle, who gave me a perfect sixty-seventh birthday party in Taos; Joan Sutherland for our long talks and the ceremonial matcha tea with accoutrements.

Deep thank-yous also to Dr. Mark Renneker, Patti Stillwell, Julia Cameron, Bill Addison, Jacqueline West, Lib O'Brien, Ruth Zaporah, Mark and Iris Keltz, Asha Greer, Seth Friedman, Caroline Albin, Vicki Buckingham, Geneen Roth and Matt Weinstein, Lorraine Ciancio, Jean Leyshon, Carol Reisen, Patrick Flanagan.

Special thanks to the acupuncturists Sandy Canzone and Sharada Hall.

Thank you to Marise Maixner for discussing endlessly the preface with me.

My darling students Dorotea Mendoza, Pam Gustafson, Bonnie Sarmiento, Armely Matas, Ryder Finnegan, Justine Kaltenbach, Sharyn Dimmick, Kevin Moul, Sarah Rauch, Carolyn Antonio, and many more: your support really helped.

Special thanks to Saundra Goldman and Sonja Lillvik for teaching the France retreat.

Thank you to David MacDonald, who put me in touch with Zhan Zhou, who helped me mightily with Chinese translations.

Thank you to Mabel Dodge Luhan House, where I wrote an early draft, and to Barbara Zaring and Stephen Rose, in whose house one December I read the final draft.

Thank you, Stella Reed, for typing the crazy-quilt handwritten manuscript with great skill and intelligence.

Much appreciation to Wendy, Susana, Michele, Eddie, Carol, John Dear, for reading earlier drafts.

Thank you to Scott Edelstein, longtime dharma pal and now agent, for his incisive discussion in helping the book's direction and who then lovingly, with clear, wise determination, placed it with Shambhala; and thank you to Jennifer Urban-Brown from Shambhala for her astute final edits, and to the whole staff at Shambhala, who seem to meet endlessly to create a beautiful product.

Beings, seen and unseen, have helped, and if I have forgotten you here, my heart has not; please forgive me.

ABOUT THE AUTHOR

NATALIE GOLDBERG is the author of fourteen books, including *Writing Down the Bones*, which has changed the way writing is taught in this country. She has led workshops and retreats for forty years nationally and internationally. She has also painted for as long as she has written. She lives in northern New Mexico. For more information, please visit nataliegoldberg.com.